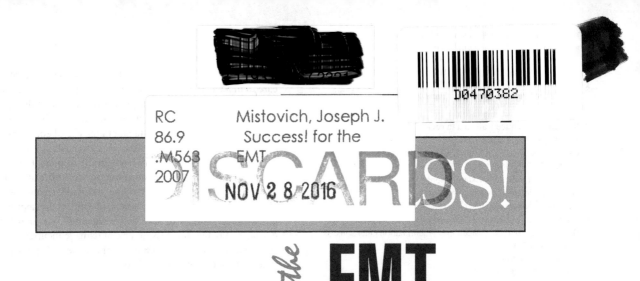

EMT

Second Edition

Complete Review

Joseph J. Mistovich, MEd, NREMT-P
Chairperson and Professor
Department of Health Professions
Youngstown State University
Youngstown, Ohio

Edward B. Kuvlesky, AAS, NREMT-P
EMS Supervisor
Indian River County Fire Rescue
Indian River County, Florida

PEARSON

Prentice
Hall

Upper Saddle River, New Jersey 07458

Library of Congress Cataloging-in-Publication Data
Mistovich, Joseph J.
   Success! for the EMT / Joseph J. Mistovich, Edward B. Kuvlesky.
      p. ; cm.
   Rev. ed. of: Prentice Hall Health review manual for the EMT-basic
self-assessment exam prep. 2003.
   Includes index.
   ISBN 0-13-225396-8
1. Emergency medicine—Examinations, questions, etc. 2. Emergency
medical technicians—Examinations, questions, etc. I. Kuvlesky,
Edward B. II. Mistovich, Joseph J. Prentice Hall Health review
manual for the EMT-basic self-assessment exam prep. III. Title.
   [DNLM: 1. Emergency Medicine—Examination Questions. WB
18.2 M678s 2007]
   RC86.9.M563 2007
   616.02'5076—dc22

2006026025

Notice: The author and the publisher of this book have taken care to make certain that the information given is correct and compatible with the standards generally accepted at the time of publication. Nevertheless, as new information becomes available, changes in treatment and in the use of equipment and procedures become necessary. The reader is advised to carefully consult the instruction and information material included in each piece of equipment or device before administration. Students are warned that the use of any techniques must be authorized by their medical adviser, where appropriate, in accord with local laws and regulations. The publisher disclaims any liability, loss, injury, or damage incurred as a consequence, directly or indirectly, of the use and application of any of the contents of this book.

Publisher: Julie Levin Alexander
Publisher's Assistant: Regina Bruno
Executive Editor: Marlene McHugh Pratt
Senior Managing Editor for Development: Lois Berlowitz
Project Manager: Sandy Breuer
Assistant Editor: Matthew Sirinides
Director of Marketing: Karen Allman
Executive Marketing Manager: Katrin Beacom
Marketing Coordinator: Michael Sirinides
Managing Editor for Production: Patrick Walsh
Production Liaison: Faye Gemmellaro
Production Editor: John Shannon, Pine Tree Composition

Manager of Media Production: Amy Peltier
New Media Project Manager: Tina Rudowski
Manufacturing Manager: Ilene Sanford
Manufacturing Buyer: Pat Brown
Senior Design Coordinator: Christopher Weigand
Cover Designer: Solid State Graphics
Interior Designer: Janice Bielawa
Composition: Pine Tree Composition
Printing and Binding: RR Donnelley
Cover Printer: RR Donnelley
Media Duplicator: ADS

Studentaid.ed.gov, the U.S. Department of Education's website on college planning assistance, is a valuable tool for anyone intending to pursue higher education. Designed to help students at all stages of schooling, including international students, returning students, and parents, it is a guide to the financial aid process. The website presents information on applying to and attending college as well as on funding your education and repaying loans. It also provides links to useful resources, such as state education agency contact information, assistance in filling out financial aid forms, and an introduction to various forms of student aid.

Pearson Education Ltd.
Pearson Education Singapore, Pte, Ltd.
Pearson Education Canada, Ltd.
Pearson Education–Japan
Pearson Education Australia Pty. Limited

Pearson Education North Asia Ltd.
Pearson Educación de Mexico. S.A. de C.V.
Pearson Education Malaysia. Pte. Ltd.
Pearson Education, Upper Saddle River, New Jersey

16   16

ISBN 0-13-225396-8

This book is dedicated to the memory of my father, who provided me with the love and encouragement that allowed me to pursue my dreams. He will always be my inspiration to continue living life to its fullest, no matter what obstacles I encounter. To my beautiful wife Andrea, who continues to be my greatest supporter and best friend. To my wonderful children, Katie, Kristyn, Chelsea, Morgan, and Kara, for helping me get through another project. Your energy, hugs, kisses, and smiles make every day so much brighter! I love you all dearly!

—Joseph J. Mistovich

To my best friends, Ed my father and Linda my wife, for their unreserved love, constant support, and unfailing encouragement to pursue my dreams of writing and inventing. To my beautiful loving children Ashley, Joshua, Matthew, and Kyle for their unconditional love, unending inspiration and childlike spiritual support, I am so proud of you all.

—Edward B. Kuvlesky

Contents

Preface

The purpose of this review manual is to help prepare you for examinations in your EMT course and your certification examination. The manual consists of a series of self-assessment sections that can identify your strengths and weaknesses in relation to the information you are studying. If you are a currently certified EMT, this manual can serve as a refresher tool or as a method to determine where your knowledge has deteriorated and which areas need specific review.

SUCCESS! for the EMT consists of multiple-choice items that include tasks found in the National Registry of EMTs 2009 Practice Analysis Test Plan. Every item has a corresponding answer and rationale.

You will also find that many of the answers and rationales are followed by page references that correspond to consistent with explanations found in Brady's Prehosptial Emergency Care 9th edition, Emergency Care 12th edition and EMT Complete textbooks, which will allow you to find more specific information on a topic or concept.

The authors and manuscript reviewers have extensive knowledge and experience as EMS educators. The items were developed in a "teacher-made test format" to allow you to test your knowledge and understanding of the material. When compiled into a series of sections, the items serve as a self-assessment tool to identify particular strengths and weaknesses in your knowledge and understanding of the information. This allows you to concentrate on specific sections that have been identified as a weakness.

This manual should be used as a tool to better prepare you for your examinations. However, there is no better preparation than studying and understanding the information that has been presented to you in your course. To best ensure your success on the examination, we encourage you to study first until you feel confident that you know the information and then use this manual as a self-assessment to determine how well you know the information. When you have identified areas of weakness, do not simply study the manual or review items. Go back and study the information presented to you, study the textbook, and use other sources to better understand the information. Once you again feel confident you know the material, retest yourself using the review manual to determine if you are better prepared for that section.

We hope this manual assists you in preparing for your examination. However, when it comes time to manage a patient in the prehospital environment, there is no time for preparation. You must draw on your existing knowledge and skills to successfully and efficiently treat the patient. Thus, it is imperative to good patient care that you are truly prepared not only to pass that examination but to take care of each and every patient you encounter to the best of your ability. Good luck in your EMS endeavors!

Joseph J. Mistovich
Edward B. Kuvlesky

Reviewers

We would like to thank the following reviewers for their comments and suggestions, which have been helpful in ensuring the accuracy and clarity of questions.

Chief Andy Baillis, EMT-P
Rittman EMS
Rittman, OH
EMS Instructor
Wayne County Schools Career Center
Smithville, OH

Captain Robin M. Broxterman, FF/EMT-P
Fire and EMS Instructor
Colerain Township Department of Fire and EMS
Great Oaks Joint Vocational Schools
Cincinnati, OH

James S. Lion, Jr., AEMT-I
EMS Lieutenant
Williamsville Fire Department
Erie County EMS Instructor
Williamsville, NY

Rick Puckett, NREMT-P, BS
Assistant Education Coordinator
Boyle County EMS
Danville, KY

Introduction

ABOUT THE SUCCESS! SERIES

SUCCESS! is a complete review system that combines relevant exam-style questions with a self-assessment format to provide you with the best preparation for your exam.

- Build your experience and exam confidence!
- Practice with realistic exam-style questions.

The SUCCESS! program is a complete method for increasing pass rates in many health professions from EMS to Nursing Assisting. We invite you to use our exam preparation system and HAVE SUCCESS!

Prentice Hall's complete SUCCESS! system includes review for the following areas:

Clinical Laboratory Science/
  Medical Technology
Dental Assisting
Dental Hygiene
Emergency Medical Services
Health Information Management

Massage Therapy
Medical Assisting
Nursing Assisting
Pharmacy Technician
Phlebotomy
Surgical Technology

ABOUT SUCCESS! FOR THE EMT

Prentice Hall is pleased to present *SUCCESS! for the EMT* as part of a review series on the various EMS education levels. The authoritative text gives you expert help in preparing for certifying examinations.

ABOUT THE BOOK

SUCCESS! for the EMT, by Joseph J. Mistovich and Edward B. Kuvlesky, has been designed to help students prepare for the written course and certification exams. It can also be used as a review for currently certified EMTs. More than 1,000 multiple-choice items reflect assessment, management and pathophysiology related to common tasks performed by the EMT. The multiple-choice items are similar to those found on teacher-made exams and certifying exams. Working through these items will help you assess your strengths and weaknesses in each section.

- **Answers and Rationales:** Correct answers and comprehensive rationales are provided to assist you in better understanding each item. Rationales are presented so that you may also learn why answers that you incorrectly gave are wrong. Many of the answers and rationales can be referenced directly to Brady's *Prehospital Emergency Care*, *Emergency Care*, and *EMT Complete* textbooks where supporting information can be found.
- **EMT Self-Assessment Practice Test:** An EMT-Basic comprehensive self-assessment test is provided as a practice exam to test your overall knowledge of the information.

ABOUT THE CD-ROM:

A CD-ROM is included in the back of this book. The accompanying CD includes 150 multiple-choice questions for extra practice. A glossary of words and definitions is included to help you review the necessary terminology.

BRADY WEBSITE FOR ADDITIONAL RESOURCES

Visit our website at www.bradybooks.com for links to related educational resources. You will want to bookmark this site and return frequently for the most current information about Brady texts and online offerings as you continue on your path to success.

Study Tips

So, you're getting ready for an exam. Congratulations for making it to this point. Now let's help you make the next step—doing your best on this exam. Some people find test taking unsettling, unnerving, and even scary! Use this book as an opportunity to practice physical preparation, information review, and exam techniques.

PHYSICAL PREPARATION

The key to maximizing your potential on a test is to be at your personal best. Along with mental preparation, physical preparation should be included in a good study strategy. Physical preparation includes getting adequate rest and exercising. It also includes eating a balanced meal the night before and the morning of the exam. Your brain works best when it has access to a supply of glucose. So fruits, grains, vegetables, and pasta are important foods. Try to avoid caffeine and foods with high sugar content on the morning of the exam. These foods provide a short burst of energy, but when they are used up, the slump will significantly reduce your ability to function.

Try some physical exercise the days before the exam, although not to the point of exhaustion. Increasing cardiovascular perfusion will also increase perfusion to the brain. More oxygen circulating in the brain can only be good, right? Exercise is also an outlet for stress, making it easier to get a good night's sleep.

INFORMATION REVIEW

Contrary to popular belief, preparing for an exam should not include extensive last-minute studying. You've been studying for months, you know the material, and cramming now will probably cause an intellectual shutdown. Review the material for short periods of time and take frequent breaks. Try study groups of three to five people for review; the active discussion will be an excellent way to reinforce the material and retain the information.

While knowing the material is essential, physical preparation is equally important. Remember, review only in brief intervals, use a study group, and don't cram.

TAKING THE EXAMINATION

An exam is not written by happenstance; it's an art and a science. Each time you take an exam, it's a chance to evaluate your knowledge as well as master the test-taking process. Exams are generally built to measure *minimum* competency. Certification or recertification exams are usually not designed to test total knowledge, ability to expertly function in the field, or even your level of professionalism. They are an attempt to evaluate your reading comprehension and judgment.

There are two basic kinds of questions found on most certification exams—multiple choice and true/false. Each question is built in a specific way to test your ability and your knowledge. Knowing how the questions are constructed may help you during the exam.

Multiple-choice questions consist of two parts: stems and answers. A stem is the actual question part, and the list of answers that follows contains one correct answer and several distracters. Distracters are designed to (what else?) distract you from the correct response. Multiple-choice questions require you to use knowledge, judgment, and expertise to answer the question. Use the process of elimination.

When answering a multiple-choice question, read the question and all the answers first. Then begin the process of elimination, starting with the most obvious incorrect answer and sorting your way through until you're left with one or two possible answers. Got a problem picking from those? Then reread the stem. If it would make it easier, rephrase the question looking for key words that give you a hint about the answer. Don't forget to look at the grammar—is the stem in plural form or singular? Whatever process you use, try not to spend more than two minutes on any one question.

You may find a topic is covered in several consecutive questions. In this case, be sure all your answers are similar and seem to fit together. It might be helpful to use the previous answers to validate each new set of choices. Another option is to check the next question because sometimes the answer, or a strong hint to one question, is the stem of the following question. Remember, when reading multiple-choice responses, the correct answer may be the most comprehensive choice—the one that combines several of the other answers or includes more details.

If the exam contains true/false questions, remember that statements containing absolute terms, like *never, always,* and *only,* will usually be false. Very little of medicine, or life itself, is absolute. Statements that contain words like *maybe* or *sometimes* tend to be true.

The scientific part of test building is putting all the information into questions, and it is an art form in the way the questions are put together to evaluate you. The key is to read each question carefully—try not to scan because you miss important key words like *incorrect* or *not* that would cause you to waste time or, more important, miss the answer. Remember your all-important "three Ps": be prudent, pace yourself, and use patience.

WRAPPING UP

You know how people say to go with your first hunch? Well, they're right. Your brain makes immediate connections based on stored information and your experience. Don't be afraid that the answer is wrong just because you didn't go through all the usual steps of logic. Research shows that first impressions tend to be correct.

It's okay to choose the same letter answer two or three times in a row. The answers are put into a question at random, so it could be that the same letter shows up as being correct up to five times. Don't change your answer if you have chosen the same letter more than once.

You have done the best you can by participating in class, practicing your skills, and reading your material. Trying to teach yourself the curriculum at the last minute just won't work, and ultimately your patients will suffer. Trust yourself and you abilities. Practice some of the tips in this section as your proceed through this book, and in the days before the exam, remember to eat well, exercise, and get plenty of sleep.

KEYS TO SUCCESS ACROSS THE BOARDS

- Study, Review, and Practice
- Keep a positive, confident attitude
- Follow all directions on the examination
- Do your best

Good luck!

Please visit http://www.prenhall.com/success for additional tips on studying, test taking, and other keys to success. At this stage of your education and career, you will find these tips helpful.

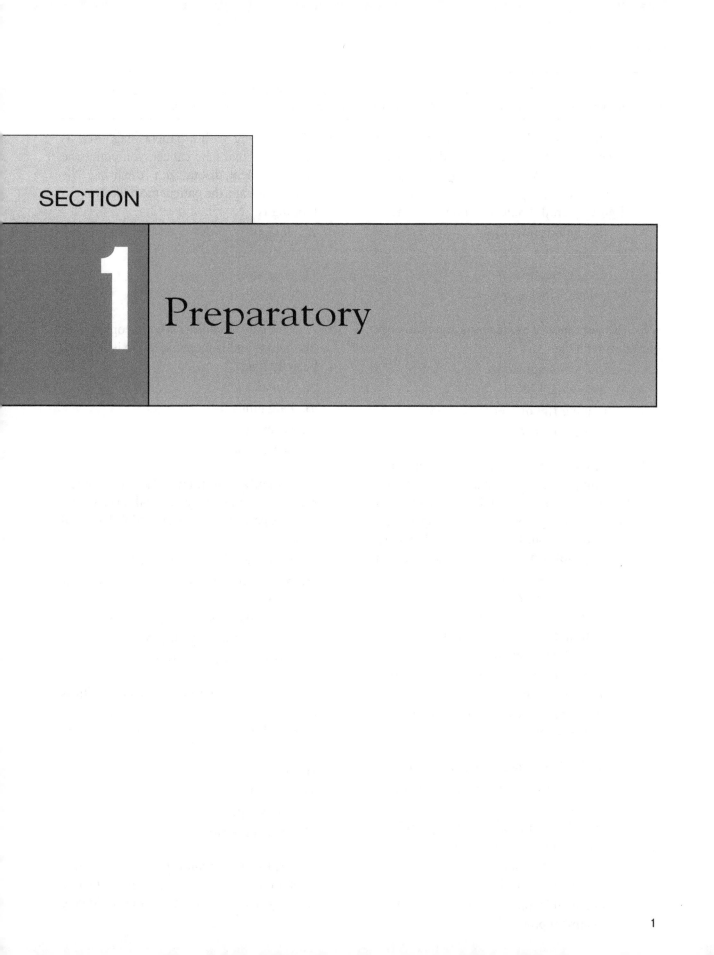

SECTION

1

Preparatory

DIRECTIONS Each of the questions or incomplete statements below is followed by suggested answers or completions. Select the **one answer** that is best in each case.

1. Which of the following is not one of the components of an EMS system identified by the "Technical Assistance Program Assessment Standards" provided by the National High-way Traffic Safety Administration?

   A. regulation and policy

   B. equipment

   C. communications

   D. resource management

2. The assurance of a safe rescue operation begins with the:

   A. incident commander.

   B. individual EMT.

   C. ranking fire officer.

   D. scene safety officer.

3. You arrive on the scene of a shooting in a housing project and find a patient lying on the sidewalk in a pool of blood. An obvious large gaping open wound to the upper thigh is spurting blood. The patient is still clutching a pistol while thrashing around and screaming. Your first action should be to:

   A. immediately apply direct pressure to the open thigh wound.

   B. restrain the patient and attempt to control the weapon.

   C. retreat and clear the bystanders from around the patient.

   D. attempt to knock the gun from the patient's hand.

4. Medical direction in an EMS system is:

   A. provided by a supervising emergency nurse.

   B. provided by the employing agency's training or education staff.

   C. the ultimate responsibility of a physician medical director.

   D. provided by the use of well-defined treatment protocols.

5. When dealing with a patient diagnosed as having terminal lung cancer, you notice the patient is silent, distant, and despairing. The emotional stage the patient most likely is exhibiting is:

   A. denial.

   B. bargaining.

   C. acceptance.

   D. depression.

6. A terminally ill patient who is coping with his disease and is prepared to die is likely to be exhibiting:

   A. denial.

   B. bargaining.

   C. acceptance.

   D. depression.

7. Your family and friends lack the understanding of emergency medical services and your responsibilities as an EMT. This will most likely:

   A. lead to a stressful relationship.

   B. relieve them of undue worry while you are working.

   C. lessen their frustrations with the requirements of your job.

   D. reduce their fear of separation.

8. A version of Critical Incident Stress Debrief-ing that is held within one to four hours following a critical incident is called a(n):

   A. review.

   B. defusing.

   C. follow up.

   D. incident recap.

9. You are treating a trauma patient with a large laceration to his upper extremity that is spurting blood. Which of the following

body substance isolation equipment is not necessary for protection in this situation?

A. eyewear with side shields.

B. latex gloves.

C. face mask vinyl gloves.

D. a HEPA respirator.

10. Your legal right to function as an EMT is contingent upon:

A. acquiring medical direction.

B. maintaining malpractice insurance.

C. mastery of the necessary skills.

D. acting in an ethical manner.

11. Permission must be obtained prior to rendering care to a patient. This is termed:

A. consent.

B. an "acknowledgment of care."

C. EMS treatment recognition.

D. a precare protocol.

12. You arrive on the scene and find lying on the street corner a 45-year-old patient who responds to your questions with inappropriate words and phrases. You should:

A. immediately assess your patient and initiate emergency care.

B. attempt to determine the patient's name, address, and phone number.

C. contact the police and wait for their consent to initiate care.

D. assume that the words indicate expressed consent and begin treatment.

13. Which patient is most likely capable of refusing treatment?

A. a patient who grabs your arm when obtaining consent

B. a patient who is under the influence of alcohol

C. a patient who gestures you away when obtaining consent

D. a patient who speaks with inappropriate words

14. You are assessing a 62-year-old female patient who complains of chest pain and refuses transport. Her husband requests that you transport her. You initiated treatment prior to her refusing transport. Given these circumstances, you should:

A. continue treatment and begin transport.

B. cease additional treatment and gain written permission from her husband.

C. immediately re-evaluate her level of competency.

D. transport her and then contact medical control for additional assistance.

15. A patient refuses treatment. She is alert and oriented and answers questions appropriately. She refuses to sign a Release from Liability Form. Your best action would be to:

A. have both you and your partner sign for the patient.

B. leave the scene and have your partner sign as a witness to the refusal.

C. leave the scene quickly and advise the husband to call back if needed.

D. have the husband sign the form as a witness to the wife's refusal.

16. A patient continues to refuse treatment or transport after assessment and explanation of the consequences of refusing care and transport. Prior to departing the scene, you should:

A. say nothing and avoid any eye contact with the family and patient.

B. try again to persuade the patient to accept treatment and transport.

C. prepare to transport the patient in spite of his repeated refusals.

D. describe complications of refusal to the patient, using the appropriate medical terminology.

17. You transport a patient to an emergency department that is extremely busy. The ward clerk yells out to move the patient to any of the rooms that are empty. While you and your partner move the patient to a hospital bed, you are toned out for another emergency. On your way out of the emergency department, you can find only the ward clerk to tell that the patient is in room 2A. You then respond to your next call. This action could result in:
    A. a continuous quality improvement investigation for improper consent.
    B. a charge of abandonment by the patient you just transported.
    C. a charge of negligence by the patient to whom you are responding.
    D. better continuation of care delivered by the emergency department.

18. A woman contacts you and states that she is the grandmother of a minor patient you transported. She requests information related to the assessment findings and care of the patient. She states she is the patient's legal guardian. The best action for you to take is:
    A. to provide the information requested and document the conversation.
    B. to provide the information, but there is no need to document the conversation.
    C. to provide the information and then contact your supervisor.
    D. not to release the information until a release form is obtained.

19. Your patient has a deformity to the midshaft of the forearm. You choose to check the radial pulse. In relation to the deformity, this pulse would be considered:
    A. proximal.
    B. transverse.
    C. lateral.
    D. distal.

20. The term *dorsal* refers to which part of the body?
    A. front
    B. side
    C. back
    D. top

21. To place the patient in a Fowler's position, you would position him:
    A. lying face up with the upper body elevated at a 45 to 60 degree angle.
    B. lying on his left or right side with his legs elevated 45 to 60 degrees.
    C. lying face up with his lower body elevated 12 inches.
    D. lying face up with the upper body elevated 15 degrees.

22. Away from or being the farthest from a point of origin is referred to as:
    A. distal.
    B. proximal.
    C. deep.
    D. superficial.

23. The midaxillary line is located at the center of:
    A. the sole of the foot.
    B. each collarbone.
    C. the armpit.
    D. the anterior chest.

24. The term *bilateral* refers to:
    A. both lungs.
    B. one side.
    C. frontal skull.
    D. both sides.

25. Which of the following would not be considered a baseline vital sign?
    A. breathing
    B. breath sounds
    C. capillary refill
    D. skin, color, temperature, and condition

26. You are assessing a 58-year-old female complaining of shortness of breath. You find minimal movement of the chest during inhalation and exhalation. You would best describe this characteristic as:
    A. labored.
    B. shallow.
    C. retractive.
    D. noisy.

27. While assessing a 25-year-old male patient who was involved in a motor vehicle crash, you note unequal pupils. This sign likely indicates that the patient is possibly suffering from:
    A. hypoperfusion.
    B. a head injury.
    C. inadequate breathing.
    D. a chest injury.

28. Pupils should be assessed for:
    A. location, constriction, and equality.
    B. size, equality, and symmetry.
    C. equality and reactivity.
    D. size, equality, and reactivity to light.

29. Unequal pupils can be an indication of:
    A. drug use.
    B. cardiac arrest.
    C. stroke.
    D. hypoxia.

30. Which of the following is a symptom?
    A. abdominal pain
    B. retractions
    C. bleeding from the forehead
    D. hot skin temperature

31. While lifting a patient from the ground, your back should be:
    A. curved slightly outward and not locked.
    B. curved slightly inward in a locked-in position.

C. in a relaxed position of comfort.
    D. parallel to the ground and in a locked-in position.

32. Which technique best protects your back from injury when carrying a heavy object?
    A. When lifting, lift with a twisting motion.
    B. Hyperextend your back by leaning backward.
    C. Keep the weight as close to your body as possible.
    D. Keep your back in a relaxed unlocked position.

33. Your patient, who is alert and oriented and has no critical illness or injury, is on the second floor of his house in the back bedroom. The best possible method to move the patient down the steps to the ground floor is by:
    A. securing the patient in a seated position in a stair chair.
    B. using the stretcher with the carriage in the up position.
    C. securing the patient to a long backboard with immobilization straps.
    D. carrying the patient using a two-person extremity lift.

34. To help prevent injury when performing a one-handed carrying technique, you should refrain from:
    A. keeping your abdominal muscles tight.
    B. bending at the hips but try to bend at the waist.
    C. positioning your back in a locked-in position.
    D. leaning to the opposite side excessively.

35. The preferred method to move a responsive, noninjured patient down steps is by the use of a:
    A. long spine board.
    B. ambulance stretcher.
    C. stair chair.
    D. vest type immobilization device.

36. Which of the following is correct and should be used to aid against injury when performing a logroll?
    A. Use your shoulder muscles whenever possible.
    B. Lean toward the patient from your waist, not your hips.
    C. Use your lower back muscles to support your weight.
    D. Keep your back in a relaxed position by leaning back.

37. Whenever possible when moving an object, you should:
    A. push it rather than pull it.
    B. lift it from the waist.
    C. pull it as low as possible to the ground.
    D. lift it as far from the body as possible.

38. In which of the following situations would an emergency move of a patient be appropriate?
    A. to shield him from curious onlookers (protect modesty)
    B. to gain access to another patient who is critically injured
    C. so law enforcement officers can direct traffic through the scene
    D. the patient complains of neck pain with numbness

39. You arrive on the scene and find a 34-year-old male patient lying in a hospital bed in his home. The dispatcher notifies you that the patient is HIV positive and has AIDS. When you arrive at the scene, his sister greets you at the door. She informs you that the patient is coughing up blood-tinged sputum, has been sweating at night profusely, and has lost weight recently. Your next immediate action should be to:
    A. refuse to enter the scene because of your risk of contracting HIV.
    B. put on gloves, eye protection, and a HEPA respirator before entering.
    C. apply a surgical mask to the patient to reduce the risk of droplet spread.
    D. contact medical direction to determine whether you should enter the scene.

40. You arrive on the scene and find a 20-year-old male patient who was involved in an auto crash. Upon your assessment, you note that the patient cannot tell you what date it is, where he is, or whom he is with. The patient refuses to let you examine him further and refuses any emergency care. You should:
    A. have the patient sign a refusal form and then leave the scene.
    B. turn the patient over to the police on the scene and then leave.
    C. begin to administer emergency care to the patient and then transport him, using restraints if necessary.
    D. have the police place the patient under protective custody so that you can administer emergency care.

41. You and your partner Mim are treating a 50-year-old male with a history of diabetes. Your patient is complaining of a severe headache that started approximately an hour ago. Mim obtains vital signs and places the patient on the pulse oximeter. He quickly notices that the heart rate is 40 beats per minute. He states that he palpated a radial

pulse of 84 beats per minute. What does this discrepancy in pulse rates likely indicate?

A. The pulse oximeter is relatively new technology and may have inaccurate readings.

B. The pulse oximeter is not accurately reading the blood flow and oxygen saturation.

C. The diabetic patient's pulse rate may vary greatly, which is a common sign of this disease.

D. Your partner has made a grave error while obtaining the patient's pulse rate, which requires you to re-evaluate the pulse rate.

42. You and your partner suspect the patient could be hypoxic. Which of the following conditions may produce an inaccurate pulse oximeter reading?

A. hyperthermia

B. hypertension

C. hypoglycemia

D. hypoperfusion

✓answers & rationales

1.

B. Equipment is not one of the recommended standards identified by the Technical Assistance Program Assessment Standards. The ten standards are regulation and policy, resource management, human resources and training, transportation, facilities, communications, public information and education, medical direction, trauma systems, and evaluation.

2.

B. Each individual is responsible for his own personal safety. Other rescuers have specific responsibilities for ensuring a safe rescue operation by observing for unsafe activities. This does not relieve the EMT from the responsibility of ensuring personal safety at all times.

3.

C. Personal safety is your primary role and responsibility, while safety of the crew, patient, and bystander is your second priority. Once safety is ensured, the patient's needs become your first priority.

4.

C. The physician medical director of an EMS system is responsible for all patient care and clinical aspects of system management. The other individuals listed in the question play roles in medical direction, although they do not assume ultimate responsibility.

5.

D. The patient could display five various emotional stages associated with death and dying. Depression is associated with silent, distant, sad, and despairing behavior.

6.

C. Acceptance is when the patient appears to accept death. He typically is no longer afraid to die.

7.

A. Your family's and friends' lack of understanding of your role and responsibility as an EMT will likely lead to a stressful relationship with them. Other stress responses by family and friends can include fear of separation or of being ignored, worry about on-call situations, frustration with the inability to plan, and frustration with your desire to share your experiences.

8.

B. A formal CISD is held within 24 to 72 hours after a critical incident. A team of peer counselors guides rescuers through varied phases of discussion. Defusing is a version of CISD that is held within 1 to 4 hours following a critical incident. Those directly involved in the incident attend the defusion.

9.

D. A high efficiency particulate air (HEPA) respirator or N-95 mask is used to filter out the organism responsible for transmitting tuberculosis. Unless your patient is exhibiting signs and symptoms of tuberculosis, there is no need to wear a HEPA respirator. Vinyl or latex gloves, eye wear with side shields, face mask, and gowns are appropriate to wear when contact with spurting blood or splashes is suspected.

10.

A. Your legal right to function as an EMT is contingent upon acquiring medical direction through protocols and standing orders. Without medical direction, you cannot function. It is an ethical responsibility to strive to achieve mastery of your skills.

11.

A. *Consent* is the permission to care for a patient. It must be obtained from all patients prior to treatment. There are three primary forms of consent: expressed, implied, and consent to treat a minor or mentally incompetent adult.

12.

A. Based on the concept of implied consent, you should immediately assess your patient and initiate emergency care.

13.

C. A competent adult has the right to refuse treatment. A patient with an altered mental status or under the influence of alcohol or drugs may be considered incompetent. Incompetency depends upon the extent to which the drugs or alcohol are clouding the patient's judgment. Orally refusing or taking other actions (such as gesturing) that imply refusal are considered valid forms of patient refusal.

14.

C. When dealing with refusal issues, determining the patient's competency or lack of competency is important. A competent adult has the right to refuse treatment or to withdraw from treatment once it has started.

15.

D. The best answer is to have the patient's husband sign as a witness to the refusal. The witnessed refusal form becomes a part of the legal documentation of the patient's refusal. You must document all aspects of the patient encounter to include history obtained and physical exam findings. Also, document your attempts at treatment and transport.

16.

B. Before leaving any patient who has refused treatment or transport, always try one last time to persuade the patient to accept emergency care and transport.

17.

B. Termination of care without ensuring the proper continuation of care by a competent practitioner can result in a charge of abandonment. In the hospital, proper transfer of care to an equally or higher qualified health care practitioner must occur. Failure to properly transfer that care can result in a charge of abandonment.

answers & rationales

18.

D. Releasing confidential information requires a written release form signed by the patient or a legal guardian. Do not release confidential information about the patient to someone claiming to be a legal guardian. Guardianship must be established.

19.

D. *Distal* is best described as distant from the point of reference. In most cases, the point farthest from the heart could be referred to as distal. In this case, the radial pulse is away from the heart and from the midshaft deformity, the point of reference.

20.

C. *Dorsal* refers to the back of the body. *Posterior* and *dorsal* have the same meaning; however, posterior is a more commonly used descriptive anatomical term.

21.

A. The Fowler's position places the patient supine, on his back, with his upper body elevated at a 45 to 60 degree angle. The Trendelenburg position places the patient supine with his legs elevated 12 inches.

22.

A. *Distal* is distant or away from the point of reference.

23.

C. The midaxillary line extends from the middle of the armpit to the ankle. It is used as an anatomical point of reference.

24.

D. *Bilateral* refers to the patient's right and left or both sides.

25.

B. Breath sounds are assessed as part of the focused history and physical exam and are not considered a component of the baseline vital signs. Capillary refill, usually more accurate in infants and young children, is considered a vital sign.

26.

B. Shallow breathing is characterized by slight movement of the chest or abdomen during breathing. It is an indication that very little volume of air is moving in and out of the lungs. It is considered to be a sign of inadequate breathing. Positive pressure ventilation must be initiated when the breathing is shallow.

27.

B. Unequal pupils can indicate a head injury, stroke, or artificial eye. Usually, one pupil is also fixed or not reacting to light. Hypoxia and hypoperfusion can cause the pupils to become sluggish but not unequal. Chest injury is most likely to cause hypoxia resulting in sluggish pupils.

28.

D. Pupils should be assessed for three factors: size, equality, and reactivity to light.

29.

C. Unequal pupils can indicate a stroke or head injury. Don't overlook the possibility that the patient has an artificial eye.

30.

A. A sign is something you can observe. You can see retractions, you can see bleeding, and you can feel skin temperature. Abdominal pain is a condition that cannot be observed, and it must be described by the patient. This is known as a *symptom*.

31.

B. When lifting a patient, the back should be kept in a locked-in position that naturally forces an inward curve.

32.

C. Try to carry objects as close to your body as possible to prevent injury. Refrain from lifting and twisting at the same time. Keep your back locked in a natural position, not hyperextended.

33.
A. When possible and if medically appropriate, use a stair chair to move the patient down stairs. Typically, it is too difficult to maneuver the stretcher up and down steps. An extremity lift is used only to place the patient onto a device to move him.

34.
D. When carrying an object with one hand, you should avoid leaning too far to the opposite side. Keeping your back in a locked-in position by keeping your abdominal muscles tight will help to prevent this unnatural position. When bending, you should bend at the hips, not at the waist.

35.
C. The preferred method is to use a stair chair, which is used for the responsive patient who does not have a spinal injury. Using a stair chair will reduce the potential for EMT lifting injuries.

36.
A. When performing the logroll technique, try to use your stronger shoulder muscles rather than your weaker back muscles. Support your body with your free hand, not your back muscles. When leaning toward the patient, try to lean at the hip, not the waist.

37.
A. Always push the object if possible. You are less apt to sustain an injury.

38.
B. You should use an emergency move only if there is an immediate danger to the patient or rescuer or to gain access to a critically injured patient. Moving the first patient to gain access to a second patient that needs immediate life-saving treatment is correct.

39.
B. The patient is displaying signs of possible tuberculosis infection, such as blood-tinged sputum, night sweats, and weight loss. Also, he is at higher risk for TB infection due to his HIV status. You should put on gloves and eye protection as a normal routine of body substance isolation protection as well as a HEPA respirator or a N-95 mask. The HEPA respirator or N-95 mask will block out the very small TB bacteria and prevent the transmission of the disease to you. If you are using a HEPA respirator that does not have an exhalation valve, you also can place one on the patient to reduce the incidence of a respiratory droplet transmission.

40.
C. The patient has an altered mental status and is disoriented to time, place, and person. At this point, he is unable to make a rational decision and should be treated based on implied consent. If necessary, restrain the patient and provide emergency care.

41.
B. A pulse rate reading on the pulse oximeter that does not correspond with the patient's actual pulse rate is an indication that the pulse oximeter is not accurately reading the blood flow and oxygen saturation. To rectify this problem, try repositioning the probe or check for impediment such as nail polish. If you are unsure whether the reading is accurate, it is important to reevaluate your findings.

42.
D. Hypoperfusion or shock could likely produce an inaccurate reading or no reading from the pulse oximeter. Other conditions that also produce erroneous readings are hypothermia, cold injury to the extremities, excessive movement, seizures, nail polish, carbon monoxide poisoning, and anemia.

2

Airway, Respiration, and Ventilation

DIRECTIONS Each of the questions or incomplete statements below is followed by suggested answers or completions. Select the **one answer** that is best in each case.

1. The epiglottis:
   A. closes shut over the trachea during inhalation.
   B. opens the esophagus during exhalation.
   C. blocks the opening of the trachea during swallowing.
   D. keeps air from entering the esophagus during ventilation.

2. The cricoid cartilage is located:
   A. in the superior portion of the larynx.
   B. lateral to the larynx.
   C. at the bifurcation of the trachea.
   D. in the inferior portion of the larynx.

3. Which range of respiratory rates typically indicates the normal breathing rate for a six-year-old child?
   A. 8 to 12 times a minute
   B. 12 to 20 times a minute
   C. 15 to 30 times a minute
   D. 25 to 50 times a minute

4. Which patient is breathing adequately?
   A. eight-year-old child breathing 12 times a minute with slight chest and abdominal rise with inhalation
   B. three-month-old infant breathing 40 times a minute with obvious abdominal movement
   C. 22-year-old person breathing 26 times a minute with excessive chest rise with each breath
   D. 61-year-old person breathing 42 times a minute with a history of smoking

5. A sign of inadequate breathing in an infant is:
   A. a respiratory rate of 25 to 50 per minute.
   B. a "seesaw" breathing motion.
   C. a regular respiratory pattern.
   D. the abdomin moves with the chest wall.

6. If you are uncertain whether a patient is breathing adequately during your initial assessment, you should:
   A. immediately begin positive pressure ventilation.
   B. re-evaluate the patient's respiratory status after a few minutes.
   C. administer a high concentration of oxygen by nonrebreather mask.
   D. count the patient's respirations carefully over at least 1 minute.

7. A patient with retractions above the clavicles, between the ribs, to the notch above the sternum, and below the rib cage, is most likely showing signs of:
   A. adequate breathing with tachypnea.
   B. bradypnea with a full tidal volume.
   C. adequate breathing but with an agonal pattern.
   D. labored breathing on inhalation.

8. You note a snoring sound upon assessing the airway in an unresponsive patient who is found lying in bed. You should:
   A. place the patient on a nonrebreather mask at 15 lpm.
   B. tilt the head back and lift the chin forward.
   C. begin positive pressure ventilation with a pocket mask.
   D. assess to determine whether a carotid pulse is present.

9. When performing a maneuver on an infant to open the airway, the head should be:
   A. hyperextended to allow better movement of the tongue.
   B. kept in a neutral position or slightly extended.
   C. flexed forward to avoid kinking the trachea.
   D. maximally extended with the shoulders elevated.

10. You find a 20-year-old female who has fallen from a second story window positioned supine on the ground with her head and neck hyperextended from the fall. You should open the airway by:
    A. leaving the head and neck in the position found and perform a head-tilt, chin-lift maneuver.
    B. maintaining the hypertension of the head and perform a jaw thrust maneuver.
    C. turning the head to the side in case there is blood in the mouth.
    D. bringing the head and neck into a neutral inline position and performing a jaw-thrust maneuver.

11. The preferred method to manually open the airway of an infant when no spinal injury is suspected is the:
    A. head-tilt, chin-lift with the head and neck placed in a hyperextended position.
    B. jaw-thrust maneuver with the head and neck in a neutral position.
    C. head-tilt, chin-lift while keeping the head and neck as close to a neutral position as possible.
    D. jaw-thrust maneuver with the neck in a hyperextended position.

12. You are treating a six-year-old who fell down the cellar steps. He is unresponsive and has no gag reflex. You should perform a:
    A. jaw-thrust maneuver with padding placed under the head.
    B. head-tilt, chin-lift and insert an oropharyngeal airway.
    C. head-tilt, neck-lift and insert a nasopharyngeal airway.
    D. jaw-thrust maneuver and insert an oropharyngeal airway.

13. When at the head of a patient with a spinal injury and performing the jaw-thrust maneuver, the EMT's elbows should:
    A. rest on the patient's forehead to allow for the proper extension of the jaw.
    B. remain at least 6 inches above the surface upon which the patient is lying.
    C. remain on the surface on which the patient is lying for support.
    D. be cradled securely on the rescuer's abdomen.

14. The jaw-thrust maneuver opens the airway by:
    A. displacing the mandible and tongue forward.
    B. displacing the tongue forward by hyperextending the head.
    C. allowing the tongue to move completely into the posterior pharynx.
    D. applying backward pressure on the cricoid cartilage.

15. You are preparing to suction blood from the mouth of a 21-year-old patient. What catheter should be used?
    A. soft
    B. rigid
    C. French
    D. bulb

16. After opening the mouth to assess the airway of a trauma patient during your initial assessment, you note a large amount of blood in the oropharynx. Your next immediate action should be to:
    A. suction the blood from the mouth.
    B. apply a nonrebreather mask and administer oxygen at 15 lpm.
    C. begin ventilating the patient with a pocket mask.
    D. assess the carotid or radial pulse.

17. Which of the following catheters and suction pressures would you select to suction the nasal passage of an infant?
    A. soft catheter at 130 to 150 mmHg
    B. rigid catheter at 80 to 120 mmHg
    C. tonsil tip catheter at 130 to 150 mmHg
    D. French catheter at 80 to 120 mmHg

18. Select the correct statement pertaining to suction equipment or the technique:
    A. French or soft catheters are inserted beyond the base of the tongue in the infant.
    B. Suction should be limited to 15 seconds in the adult and 5 seconds in the infant.
    C. Suction should be applied before the catheter is inserted into the mouth.
    D. The convex side of the rigid catheter is placed against the tongue.

19. You are preparing to use a French catheter to suction the oropharynx of a 20-year-old male. To determine the length of the catheter needed, you should measure:
    A. from the corner of the patient's mouth to the tip of the ear.
    B. from the corner of the patient's mouth to the Adam's apple.
    C. from the tip of the patient's nose to the tip of the patient's ear.
    D. from the tip of the patient's nose to the patient's cricoid cartilage.

20. You are preparing to ventilate a patient using a pocket mask. You should set the oxygen liter flow to the pocket mask at:
    A. 4 lpm.
    B. 6 lpm.
    C. 10 lpm.
    D. 15 lpm.

21. When ventilating a patient, each ventilation should be delivered over:
    A. 0.5 second.
    B. 1.0 second.
    C. 2.0 seconds.
    D. 2.5 seconds.

22. You arrive on the scene and find a patient who fell off a scaffolding from about 30 feet. Upon assessment, you find sonorous (snoring) upper airway sounds; respirations are approximately 30 per minute and shallow; a radial pulse is absent; the carotid pulse is weak and rapid at about 130 per minute; and the skin is pale, cool, and clammy. You should immediately:
    A. immobilize the patient on a spine board.
    B. apply a cervical spinal immobilization collar.
    C. stabilize the head and neck and apply a nonrebreather at 15 lpm and transport the patient.
    D. perform a jaw-thrust maneuver with in-line stabilization and begin bag-valve-mask ventilation.

23. When ventilating a patient while performing the jaw-thrust maneuver, it is necessary to:
   A. maintain a mask seal with one hand while tilting the forehead backward.
   B. keep the mandible immobilized in a neutral position.
   C. hold a mask seal while lifting the mandible forward.
   D. flex the neck forward and push the mandible backward.

24. A patient being ventilated with a bag-valve-mask device that is not connected to supplemental oxygen is receiving what percentage of oxygen with each ventilation?
   A. 16 to 18 percent
   B. 21 percent
   C. 44 percent
   D. 100 percent

25. Which of the following is a desirable feature of the bag-valve-mask device?
   A. It generates lower tidal volumes than mouth to mask.
   B. It can be used by two EMTs to reduce operator fatigue.
   C. A pop-off valve cannot be disabled.
   D. A 450 mL bag-value-mask device can be used on both adults and children.

26. You are preparing to ventilate a patient with the bag-valve-mask device. Choose the correct sequence for mask placement procedure:
   A. Place the side of the mask over the cheek and the wider part over the cleft of the chin, then lower the narrow portion over the nose.
   B. Place the wider part of the mask over the cleft of the chin; then place the narrow part over the bridge of the nose.
   C. Place the narrow part of the mask over the cleft of the chin and then the wider part over the bridge of the nose.
   D. Place the narrow part of the mask over the bridge of the nose and then the wider part over the cleft of the chin.

27. When ventilating an adult patient in cardiac arrest who has an endotracheal tube in place, you should ventilate:
   A. 10 to 12 times per minute during a pause between chest compressions.
   B. 8 to 10 times per minute without synchronization with chest compressions.
   C. every 5 seconds, interposing each ventilation between chest compressions.
   D. twice during the pause following each set of 15 compressions.

28. Ideally, ventilation with a bag-valve-mask device in the cardiac arrest patient should be performed by:
   A. one EMT holding a one-handed mask seal and squeezing the bag with one hand.
   B. two EMTs with one providing a two-handed mask seal and the other squeezing the bag with two hands.
   C. three EMTs with one providing a two-handed mask seal, one squeezing the bag with two hands, and the third providing cricoid pressure.
   D. three EMTs with one holding the head-tilt, chin-lift maneuver, one providing a two-handed mask seal, and the third squeezing the bag with two hands.

29. An indication of inadequate ventilation in an adult patient would be:
    A. the rise of the chest symmetrically with each ventilation.
    B. the slowing of the heart rate from 130 per minute to 80 per minute.
    C. the increase of abdominal movement with each delivered ventilation.
    D. the change in the pupils from dilated to midsize.

30. You arrive on the scene and find a seven-year-old patient who was pulled from a pond after being submerged for 10 minutes. The first response crew is on the scene when you arrive. The patient is being ventilated at a rate of 12 ventilations per minute by mouth to mask with supplemental oxygen set at 12 lpm. The patient remains cyanotic. You should immediately:
    A. reassess the airway and ensure adequate chest rise with each ventilation.
    B. increase the oxygen flow from 12 lpm to 15 lpm.
    C. compress the stomach in case there is gastric distention.
    D. increase the ventilation rate from 12 to 24 per minute.

31. The best method to determine whether an adequate tidal volume is being delivered with each ventilation is to:
    A. observe the chest for obvious rise with each ventilation.
    B. listen for air sounds coming from the nose or mouth while squeezing the bag.
    C. feel the bag deflate when squeezing it with each ventilation.
    D. watch for a change in the patient's color.

32. A likely cause of abdominal distention while ventilating with a bag-valve-mask device is:
    A. overinflation of the reservoir device by setting the liter flow at 15 lpm.
    B. allowing for prolonged passive exhalation after each ventilation.
    C. lack of the use of an airway adjunct while providing ventilation.
    D. delivering the ventilation over a 2.5 to 3 second period.

33. When ventilating a patient with a flow-restricted, oxygen-powered ventilation device, you must ensure that:
    A. an adequate, constant oxygen supply is available.
    B. the patient has no history of chronic obstructive lung disease to avoid the chance of producing oxygen toxicity.
    C. the device does not have a pressure relief valve so that adequate tidal volumes can be delivered.
    D. the device is connected to a flow regulator able to deliver 25 lpm.

34. When attempting to ventilate a patient with a flow-restricted, oxygen-powered ventilation device, the patient's chest does not rise. You should:
    A. increase the oxygen flow from 40 lpm to 100 lpm.
    B. occlude the pressure relief valve with your thumb.
    C. reposition the head and neck and ensure a tight mask seal.
    D. increase the ventilation time from 1 to 2 seconds.

35. When ventilating a patient with a flow-restricted, oxygen-powered ventilation device, the valve should be depressed until:
    A. the pressure relief valve opens.
    B. resistance is felt on the trigger.
    C. the chest begins to rise.
    D. the audible alarm sounds.

36. When performing mouth-to-mouth ventilation, you should:
    A. not break the seal of your mouth on the patient's face between ventilations.
    B. deliver the ventilation forcefully over less than 1 second.
    C. allow for adequate exhalation by removing your mouth between ventilations.
    D. increase your rate of ventilation because supplemental oxygen is not used.

37. While performing bag-valve-mask-to-stoma ventilation, you note minimal chest rise and feel air escaping from the mouth and nose with each ventilation. You should:
    A. pinch the nose and close the mouth and continue ventilation through the stoma.
    B. secure a mask seal over the nose and mouth, occlude the stoma, and continue ventilating the patient.
    C. apply a nonrebreather mask over the nose and mouth and administer 15 lpm of oxygen.
    D. insert a nasopharyngeal airway in the stoma and ventilate with a pediatric pocket mask.

38. During insertion of the nasopharyngeal airway, you feel slight resistance. You should:
    A. use force and rapidly insert the device.
    B. stop the insertion immediately and remove the device.
    C. insert a soft suction catheter deep into the nasopharynx and apply suction for no longer than 15 seconds.
    D. be sure that the airway is being inserted straight back into the nasopharynx and then slightly twist and turn the device as you continue the insertion.

39. You determine the proper size of an oropharyngeal airway by:
    A. measuring from the tip of the nose to the tip of the earlobe.
    B. measuring from the corner of the mouth to the tip of the earlobe.
    C. choosing the same length airway as the length of the index finger.
    D. using the size formula ([16 + the patient's age in years] ÷ 4).

40. The oropharyngeal airway is designed to:
    A. isolate the trachea and protect against aspiration of secretions, blood, and vomitus.
    B. be inserted if the patient is slightly responsive.
    C. elevate the epiglottis off the glottic opening.
    D. keep the tongue from protruding into the posterior pharynx.

41. An oropharyngeal airway should not be inserted in a:
    A. patient who responds only to verbal stimuli.
    B. patient in cardiac arrest who had vomited earlier.
    C. diabetic patient with a blood glucose level of 42 mg/dL who does not respond to painful stimuli.
    D. stroke patient who has no cough or gag reflex.

42. A nasopharyngeal airway should be lubricated with:
    A. a water-soluble lubricant.
    B. lidocaine spray or jelly.
    C. a petroleum-based lubricant.
    D. sterile saline or sterile water.

43. The method used to size the nasopharyngeal airway for the proper length is to measure from the:
    A. corner of the edge of the mouth to the tip of the nose.
    B. corner of the edge of the mouth to the tip of the earlobe.
    C. bridge of the nose to the tip of the chin.
    D. tip of the nose to the tip of the earlobe.

44. A properly sized nasopharyngeal airway should:
    A. fit snugly in the nostril with the proximal end extended 2 inches beyond the tip of the nose.
    B. fit loosely in the nostril with the distal end extended 2 inches beyond the base of the tongue.
    C. be seated firmly in the nare with the proximal flange seated against the nostril.
    D. seated tightly against the nostril with enough pressure to blanch the surrounding skin.

45. The proper steps to follow when applying a nonrebreather mask or nasal cannula to the patient is to:
    A. apply the device to the patient, attach the oxygen tubing to the flowmeter, and open the flowmeter to the desired liters per minute.
    B. attach the oxygen tubing to the flowmeter, open the flowmeter to the desired liters per minute, and apply the device to the patient.

    C. open the flowmeter and set the desired liters per minute, apply the device to the patient, attach the oxygen tubing to the flowmeter.
    D. attach the oxygen tubing to the flowmeter, apply the device to the patient, open the flowmeter and set the desired liters per minute.

46. An oxygen tank is full when the pressure gauge reads:
    A. 500 psi.
    B. 2,000 psi.
    C. 3,000 psi.
    D. 5,000 psi.

47. When using a nonrebreather mask, the oxygen flow regulator should be set at:
    A. 15 lpm.
    B. 10 lpm.
    C. 8 lpm.
    D. 6 lpm.

48. You are treating a 62-year-old patient with a history of chronic obstructive pulmonary disease (COPD). The patient states, "I can't breathe" and presents with obvious signs of hypoxia. His SpO_2 reading is 80 percent and his mental status is declining. You should apply a:
    A. nonrebreather mask with the oxygen set at 10 lpm.
    B. nonrebreather mask with the oxygen set at 15 lpm.
    C. nasal cannula with the oxygen set at 8 lpm.
    D. nasal cannula with the oxygen set at 2 lpm.

49. The preferred device to deliver oxygen to a trauma patient with adequate ventilation is a:
    A. nasal cannula at 2 lpm.
    B. nonrebreather mask at 6 to 8 lpm.
    C. nonrebreather mask at 15 lpm.
    D. nasal cannula at 6 lpm.

50. The nonrebreather mask provides high concentrations of oxygen by:

    A. using high oxygen liter flow rates.

    B. allowing the patient to rebreathe some of his exhaled gas.

    C. concentrating the oxygen in the mask, nasopharynx, and oropharynx before inhalation.

    D. drawing a majority of the volume of air from the oxygen reservoir bag for inhalation.

51. Your patient continues to refuse to keep a nonrebreather mask on, even with extensive coaching. You should next:

    A. remove the nonrebreather mask and do not agitate him with another device.

    B. remove the nonrebreather mask and apply a nasal cannula.

    C. hold the mask to his face and explain the importance of oxygen therapy.

    D. remove the mask and provide blow by oxygen with the oxygen tubing.

Scenario

Questions 52–54 refer to the following scenario:

You and your partner Wilson are enjoying a well-deserved break when you are dispatched to 8356 64th Avenue for a patient complaining of shortness of breath. While en route, you both take body substance isolation precautions. Upon your arrival, you find the scene is safe. You both enter the house to find a 35-year-old female walking around the house complaining, "I can't breathe." You have the patient sit down, and you perform an initial assessment. The patient is breathing 20 times per minute, there is good chest rise, and you feel adequate air during exhalation. Her heart rate is 102 beats per minute and her skin is pale, cool, and clammy.

52. Your first action is to:

    A. insert a nasopharyngeal airway.

    B. begin ventilation with a bag-valve-mask device.

    C. administer supplemental oxygen.

    D. determine the past medical history and current medications.

Upon further assessment, you note wheezing in all lung fields. You ask the patient if she has been prescribed a metered dose inhaler (MDI). She states, "My puffer is on the night stand." You receive an order from medical direction to administer the MDI.

53. You should expect the following side effects following administration of the MDI:

    A. bradycardia and blurred vision.

    B. hypertension and salivation.

    C. tachycardia and nervousness.

    D. hypotension and sweating.

Wilson notices that the patient is breathing faster and with increased effort. The patient's mental status has deteriorated significantly. She is using the muscles in the neck when she inhales. The chest is barely rising with each breath. You quickly auscultate the lungs and hear nothing in the lower lobes and slight wheezes in the upper lobes.

54. You should immediately:

    A. begin bag-valve-mask ventilation with supplemental oxygen connected to the device.

    B. increase the liter flow to the nonrebreather mask to 20 lpm.

    C. remove the nonreberather mask and apply a nasal cannula so the breathing is not restricted.

    D. administer another dose of the medication by the metered dose inhaler.

55. When ventilating a patient who has a pulse with a bag-valve-mask device with a reservoir that is connected to an oxygen source flowing at 15 lpm, you should deliver a tidal volume of:

   A. 10 to 15 mL/kg over 1 second.
   B. 8 to 10 mL/kg over 1 to 2 seconds.
   C. 6 to 7 mL/kg over 2 seconds.
   D. 3 to 4 mL/kg over 1 second.

answers & rationales

1.

C. The epiglottis is a cartilaginous flap of tissue that is responsible for closing the opening of the trachea during swallowing. This prevents aspiration of food or other substances into the trachea and lungs.

2.

D. The cricoid cartilage, the only completely circumferential cartilaginous ring, is located in the inferior portion of the larynx. The cricoid ring, also known as *cricoid pressure,* is the landmark to perform the Sellick maneuver.

3.

C. The typical breathing rate range for children is 15 to 30 times each minute. The typical respiratory rate for the adult is 12 to 20 times each minute. The breathing rate of an infant is typically 25 to 50 times each minute. These are average, not absolute, ranges. For example, an adult patient can have a normal respiratory rate as low as 8 to 10 times per minute and as high as 24 times per minute. Elderly patients have higher resting respiratory rates, on average 20 to 22 respirations per minute. When evaluating a respiratory rate, it is important to consider the rate in relation to the whole patient assessment.

4.

B. A three-month-old infant breathing 40 times a minute with the use of the abdominal muscles is considered normal. In infants and young children, the chest wall and the chest muscles used for breathing are immature. Thus, the child relies heavily on the diaphragm and more on the abdominal muscles to breathe. This produces more abdominal movement and less chest wall movement during normal breathing. An 8-year-old child breathing 12 times a minute is slightly slow (average range is 15 to 30 times a minute). Minimal chest rise is an indicaton that the tidal volume or the depth of breathing is low or inadequate (low air volume entering the lungs). When either the respiratory rate or tidal volume is inadequate, it is necessary to ventilate the patient. A 42-year-old person breathing 26 times a minute is breathing fast (average range is 12 to 20 times a minute), which is referred to as *tachypnea.* However, this patient also has excessive rise of the chest with inhalation, indicating a full and deep tidal volume with each breath. Patients with faster than normal respiratory rates could experience inadequate breathing when the fast respiratory rate does not allow the patient to take in an adequate tidal volume with each breath. You would see shallow breathing or minimal chest rise with each inhalation. This would be an indication to begin ventilation. A 61-year-old person breathing 42 times a minute is too fast, whether he is a smoker or not.

5.

B. A sign of inadequate breathing in an infant is a "seesaw" breathing motion. This results from the abdomen and chest moving in opposite directions during breathing. This is an indication of severe respiratory distress or respiratory failure. A respiratory rate of 25 to 50 in an infant is the average range. You should expect more abdominal movement in the infant because the respiratory muscles are immature and the diaphragm is the major muscle used in breathing. The abdomen will rise and fall simultaneously with the chest on inhalation and exhalation and will not move in an opposite direction as seen in the "seesaw" motion.

6.

A. You should begin positive pressure ventilation immediately. It is best to benefit the patient and provide ventilation. If, after a few minutes, you determine that the breathing is inadequate, you have already allowed the patient to become hypoxic for that period of time, which could have serious consequences to organs, especially the brain. However, if you begin to ventilate and later determine that the ventilation is adequate, you have not caused any harm to the patient by doing the ventilation.

7.

D. A patient with retractions above the clavicles, between and below the ribs, and above the sternum, is most likely showing signs of labored breathing. Retractions indicate that the patient is struggling to move air into the chest and lungs on inhalation, which typically results in a poor

tidal volume. *Tachypnea* is a rapid respiratory rate, and *bradypnea* is a slow respiratory rate. An *agonal respiratory pattern* can be seen in patients shortly after going into cardiac arrest or in some patients who are in respiratory arrest. The agonal pattern is associated with an extremely slow and ineffective rate of respiration.

8.

B. Snoring is an indication that the tongue is partially occluding the upper airway. Perform a head-tilt, chin-lift maneuver as a priority in establishing an airway. If the patient is suspected of having a possible spine injury, perform a jaw-thrust maneuver.

9.

B. Due to the underdeveloped structures of the upper airway in the infant, the head should be kept in a neutral position or slightly extended when performing a head-tilt, chin-lift maneuver. Hyperextending the head can actually cause the trachea to become occluded, causing an airway obstruction. Flexing the head could occlude the airway by allowing the tongue to fall forward.

10.

D. Even though the head and neck are already hyperextended from the fall, they need to be brought into a neutral in-line position to avoid further injury to the spine or spinal cord. A jaw-thrust maneuver is then performed to open the airway. Any other maneuver or method could potentially manipulate the spine and cause further injury to the patient.

11.

C. The preferred method for opening the airway of an infant without a suspected spinal injury is the head-tilt, chin-lift maneuver. It is important to remember that in the infant, the head should be placed in a neutral position or slight sniffing position. If the head is overextended in the infant or child, the trachea can become obstructed.

12.
D. This patient could have a spinal injury; thus, you should open the airway by using the jaw-thrust maneuver. An oropharyngeal airway will aid in keeping the tongue away from the oropharynx, helping to maintain an open airway. Padding is placed under the shoulders of children typically less than four years of age to bring the head and torso of the body into a neutral in-line position. In the older child and the adult, approximately 1 inch of padding is placed behind the head to establish a neutral position.

13.
C. When performing the jaw-thrust maneuver, the rescuer's elbows should be placed on the surface on which the patient is lying. This provides a solid surface to maintain spinal stabilization.

14.
A. The jaw-thrust maneuver opens the airway by displacing the mandible forward while maintaining the head in a neutral position. This lifts the tongue away from the posterior wall of the pharynx.

15.
B. A hard or rigid suction catheter—also known as a *tonsil tip, tonsil sucker,* or *Yankauer*—is the preferred catheter for performing oropharyngeal suctioning. The soft or French catheter is usually used to suction the nose or nasopharynx. If the teeth are clenched partially closed and a rigid catheter cannot be inserted, the soft suction catheter can be used to suction the oropharynx.

16.
A. Blood, vomitus, or other substances in the airway must be cleared immediately with suction. Failure to do so can lead to aspiration and severe hypoxia. It is necessary to always have your suction equipment ready for use.

17.
D. The French or soft catheter is correct when suctioning the nasal passage of an infant. When doing so, you should use low to medium suction (-80 to -120 mmHg). A rigid (tonsil tip) catheter will cause injury to the soft tissue of the nasal passage. Suctioning at a rate too high (more than 120 mmHg) can cause injury to the soft tissue of the nasal passage.

18.
B. Suctioning longer than 15 seconds in the adult and 5 seconds in the infant can cause hypoxia. The patient should be hyperoxygenated before and immediately after suctioning. Inserting the catheter beyond the base of the tongue could injure soft tissue or stimulate nerves and cause a decrease in the heart rate. Suction should be applied only after the catheter is in place. The convex side of the rigid catheter is placed against the roof of the mouth, not the tongue.

19.
A. The correct length of a French or soft catheter is determined by measuring from the corner of the patient's mouth to the tip of the ear when preparing to suction the oropharynx. If you are preparing to suction the nose or nasopharynx, you should measure from the tip of the patient's nose to the tip of the earlobe.

20.
D. When using a pocket face mask to ventilate a patient who is not breathing, the oxygen flow should be set at 15 lpm.

21.
B. When ventilating an adult, child, or infant, each ventilation should be delivered over 1.0 second. This slow ventilation helps to prevent gastric distention and subsequent aspiration.

22.

D. The sonorous (snoring) sounds indicate a partially occluded airway. Thus, a manual maneuver must be performed to immediately open the airway. A jaw-thrust maneuver is the most appropriate because of the risk of possible spinal injury. Also, the patient's breathing is inadequate due to the poor tidal volume and excessively high rate. Therefore, it is necessary to immediately begin ventilation. Manual in-line stabilization should be performed at this point until the immediate life threats to the airway and breathing have been managed effectively. A cervical spinal immobilization collar should be applied during the focused history and physical exam.

23.

C. When performing the jaw-thrust maneuver, it is necessary to displace the mandible forward while keeping the head and neck stabilized in a neutral in-line position. This procedure is most commonly used for patients with suspected spinal injuries.

24.

B. Using the bag-valve-mask device without supplemental oxygen will result in the delivery of only 21 percent oxygen, the amount found in the air we breathe. When used with supplemental oxygen at 15 lpm and an oxygen reservoir, you can deliver an oxygen concentration of nearly 95 percent.

25.

B. The bag-valve-mask (BVM) device is difficult to use and fatiguing to the operator. If possible, two EMTs should ventilate a patient. One should hold the mask on the patient's face while the other squeezes the bag. The BVM rarely is able to generate higher tidal volumes than the rescuer providing mouth to mask. A nondisabling pop-off valve is not preferred. A pop-off valve that is not disabled could lead to ineffective ventilation in some patients. A 1,000 to 1,600 mL BVM must be used to ventilate adult patients and older children. A BVM that is too small in size will deliver inadequate tidal volumes to the patient and will result in hypoxia.

26.

D. The proper sequence to place a bag-valve-mask device on a patient's face is first to place the narrow part of the mask over the bridge of the nose and then to lower the mask over the nose and mouth until the wider part meets the cleft of the chin. This sequence results in a better seal on the patient's face. If the mask does not cover the bridge of the nose and the cleft of the chin, you need to select a mask of more appropriate size.

27.

B. When ventilating an adult patient in cardiac arrest, two ventilatons should be delivered during the pause after each 15 compressions. However, if the patient has an advanced airway in place (endotracheal tube, laryngeal mask airway, or esophageal tracheal combitube), the ventilations should be delivered at a rate of 8 to 10 per minute (every 7.5 to 6 seconds) without any synchronization with chest compressions. The compressor delivers continuous chest compressions with no pause for ventilation.

28.

C. In the ideal setting, three EMTs would provide ventilation to the cardiac arrest patient. One EMT would hold the mask with two hands while maintaining a head-tilt, chin-lift maneuver. The second EMT would squeeze the bag with both hands to ensure delivery of an adequate tidal volume with each ventilation. The third EMT would provide cricoid pressure to reduce gastric insufflation and the risk of aspiration. One rescuer bag-valve-mask ventilation is discouraged because it is difficult for one rescuer to maintain an effective seal and deliver an adequate volume of ventilation.

29.

C. An increase in abdominal movement is an indication that air is being forced into the esophagus and the stomach. This could potentially result in severe gastric distention that impedes ventilation or leads to aspiration.

30.

A. The patient is not being adequately ventilated. First, reassess the airway to ensure that it is open and is not occluded by the tongue, secretions, vomitus, or other substances. Then watch for chest rise with each ventilation. If the chest does not rise with each ventilation, it could be necessary to reposition the head and neck to ensure an adequate airway and deliver a tidal volume to make the chest visibly rise with each ventilation. Increasing the ventilation rate to 24 per minute is unacceptable because the range of ventilation for a child is 12 to 20 per minute. Increasing the oxygen liter flow will not necessarily increase the delivered amount of oxygen to the patient. Never decompress the stomach unless the gastric distention impedes ventilation.

31.

A. When ventilating a patient, watch for an obvious chest rise with each ventialtion when squeezing the bag. If sounds are heard around the nose and mouth, it is likely that air is leaking past the mask, indicating an inadequate mask seal, which leads to poor ventilation. The bag should deflate with little resistance while ventilating; however, this is not the best indicator that an adequate tidal volume is being delivered. If the bag progressively becomes more difficult to squeeze, consider repositioning the head or using an airway adjunct; you should also suspect a tension pneumothorax. A change in the patient's color could provide evidence of either adequate or inadequate ventilation; however, it usually takes a long period of time to get a skin color change.

32.

D. Ventilating at too fast a rate, delivering too high a tidal volume, or providing the ventilation over a period that is less than 1 second will likely force air into the esophagus and subsequently into the stomach. During ventilation, it is essential to guide the tidal volume delivery by watching for the chest to rise with each ventilation. The ventilation should be delivered over 1 second. A longer ventilation time will lead to the delivery of excessive tidal volumes that will cause air to be forced into the esophagus and into the stomach, leading to gastric distention. Gastric distention can lessen the effectiveness of ventilation by putting upward pressure on the diaphragm, limiting its movement. Also, gastric inflation can lead to regurgitation and aspiration. To prevent air from entering the stomach, you should deliver the ventilation over 1 second, allowing the chest to rise, followed by passive exhalation.

33.

A. When preparing to use a flow-restricted, oxygen-powered ventilation device, you must ensure that an adequate oxygen supply is available. Once the oxygen source has been depleted, the device can no longer be used because it is driven completely by an oxygen source. The device must have a pressure relief valve that opens at 60 cm of water pressure to avoid overventilation and trauma to the lungs. The device should deliver a peak flow rate of 40 lpm; thus, it requires a special regulator and is not connected to the standard outlet on the flow regulator.

34.

C. The oxygen flow is delivered at a constant 40 lpm and cannot be altered. The inspiratory pressure control valve opens at 60 cm of water pressure. Increasing the ventilation time will not correct the problem if it is caused by improper head position or mask seal. If, after the head position and mask seal have been checked, the chest still does not rise, an airway obstruction must be considered.

35.

C. When a patient is being ventilated with a flow-restricted, oxygen-powered ventilation device, the valve should be depressed until the chest begins to rise. Dependence on a pressure relief valve and an audible alarm is inappropriate.

36.

C. When performing mouth-to-mouth ventilation, you should break the seal of your mouth between ventilations to allow for adequate exhalation by the patient. This also allows you to breathe an adequate volume to deliver to the patient on the next ventilation. Ventilations should not be forceful and should be delivered over a 2-second period to reduce the incidence of gastric distention.

37.

A. Air escaping from the nose and mouth while ventilating a patient through his stoma is an indication that the patient has a partial laryngectomy. You should pinch the nose and close the mouth and continue ventilation through the stoma.

38.

D. A certain amount of resistance is expected when inserting a nasopharyngeal airway. Prior to insertion, ensure that the airway is properly lubricated. Also insert the device straight back into the nasopharynx, not upward. Twisting and turning the device usually allows insertion. If excessive resistance is encountered, remove the device and try the opposite nostril.

39.

B. The proper size of an oropharyngeal airway is determined by measuring from the corner of the mouth to the tip of the earlobe. You can also measure from the center of the mouth to the bottom of the angle of the jaw. The sizing formula ([16 + the patient's age in year] ÷ 4) is used to determine the proper size of the endotracheal tube for patients over 1 year of age.

40.

D. The oropharyngeal airway does not isolate the trachea or protect the airway from aspiration of vomitus, blood, or secretions. Suction should always be available when inserting the device. You should use it only on completely unresponsive patients. Failure to do so can cause the patient to gag and vomit. The oropharyngeal airway does not extend down to the epiglottis. If it does, the airway is too long. Using an oropharyngeal airway that is too long can force the epiglottis to close over the trachea, blocking the airway. The oropharyngeal airway is designed to keep the tongue away from the posterior pharyngeal wall.

41.

A. The oropharyngeal airway must be used only on unresponsive patients who have no gag or cough reflex. If responding to painful or verbal stimuli, the patient likely will gag and possibly vomit, causing further complication of the airway.

42.

A. Prior to insertion, a nasopharyngeal airway should be lubricated with a water-soluble lubricant. Never use a petroleum-based lubricant. Lidocaine jelly or spray or saline will not provide adequate lubrication and can result in trauma to the nasopharynx upon insertion.

43.

D. To determine the proper length of a nasopharyngeal airway, measure from the tip of the nose to the tip of the earlobe.

44.

C. Blanching occurs when the nasal opening becomes white. The presence of blanching at the nasal opening indicates that the nasopharyngeal airway is too large. This is a result of blood being forced from the area from excessive pressure. The airway should be inserted until the flange is seated firmly on the nostril.

45.

B. When administering oxygen to the patient, you should first set up the oxygen delivery system. Second, prepare and attach the oxygen delivery device to the flowmeter, set the desired liter per minute flow and then apply the device to the patient. Applying a nonrebreather mask to the patient without oxygen flow can reduce the patient's tidal volume and cause or increase hypoxia.

46.

B. The best way to measure the volume in the oxygen tank, regardless of the size of tank, is to use the pressure gauge. A full tank has 2,000 psi of pressure. As the tank volume decreases, so does the pressure in the tank.

47.

A. When using a nonrebreather oxygen mask, the oxygen regulator must be set so that the reservoir on the mask remains inflated. Typically, the oxygen flow required to keep the reservoir inflated is 15 lpm.

48.

B. In the prehospital setting, always provide high flow oxygen to the COPD patient who is presenting with evidence of hypoxia. The nasal cannula will not maximize oxygenation of the patient; thus, a nonrebreather mask set at 15 lpm. A nasal cannula set at 6 lpm will deliver only up to 44 percent oxygen. Even though the patient may be on a nasal cannula at home with a flow of 2 to 3 lpm, if he is exhibiting signs and symptoms of hypoxia, it is necessary to maximize the oxygen delivery.

49.

C. The preferred prehospital device for oxygen delivery is the nonrebreather mask. It delivers about a 90 percent to 95 percent oxygen concentration. It can be used only in the patient who has an adequate respiratory rate and an adequate tidal volume. Adjust the flow meter to 15 lpm to prevent the nonrebreathing oxygen reservoir bag from completely collapsing when the patient inhales. The nasal cannula is used only when a patient is not able to tolerate a nonrebreathing mask.

50.

D. The nonrebreather mask provides high concentrations of oxygen primarily because of the oxygen reservoir bag that collects 100 percent oxygen. When the patient inhales, the majority of the tidal volume being breathed in is drawn from the reservoir bag, which is highly enriched with oxygen. Because the amount of volume in the reservoir bag directly determines the tidal volume on inhalation, it is imperative that the bag be fully inflated prior to the inhalation.

51.

B. If a patient is unable to tolerate a nonrebreather mask, you should first attempt to coach the patient. If that is not effective, remove the nonrebreather mask and apply a nasal cannula. If the patient cannot tolerate the nasal cannula, administer oxygen by the blow-by technique.

52.

C. This patient's breathing status is adequate because the respiratory rate is within a normal range, and there is good chest rise, indicating an adequate tidal volume. Because the breathing is adequate, the patient does not need to be ventilated. However, because the patient is complaining of dyspnea, you should administer supplemental oxygen to the patient. You can begin with a nasal cannula at 2 to 4 lpm and continue to titrate up to achieve the desired response from the patient and an adequate SpO2 reading of 94% or greater. If the response is not adequate and the liter flow is maximized at 6 lpm, switch to a nonrebreather mask.

53.

C. The common side effects of a beta agonist drug are tachycardia, tremors, shakiness, nervousness, dry mouth, nausea, and vomiting. It is important to explain these common side effects to your patient prior to administering the drug. Explaining the common side effects will help to reduce the patient's stress and apprehension.

54.

A. The patient's breathing has deteriorated from adequate to inadequate. You should immediately provide positive pressure ventilation with the bag-valve-mask ventilation and supplemental oxygen. Administering high flow oxygen will not help this patient because her tidal volume is inadequate.

55.

A. A tidal volume of 10 mL/kg to 15 mL/kg delivered over a 1-second period should be delivered when providing ventilation by bag-valve-mask device or mouth to mask to a patient with a pulse. A smaller tidal volume will be used for the patient in cardiac arrest.

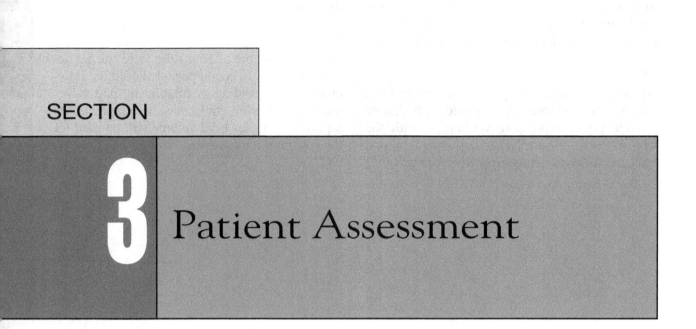

SECTION

3 Patient Assessment

DIRECTIONS Each of the questions or incomplete statements below is followed by suggested answers or completions. Select the **one answer** that is best in each case.

1. Scene safety begins:
   A. when you have reached the patient's side.
   B. just prior to reaching the patient's side so the patient will not be distracted when you perform the primary assessment.
   C. as you are arriving at the scene and before even exiting the ambulance.
   D. as you approach the scene once you have exited the ambulance.

2. Scenes that are most likely to result in injury to an EMT involve:
   A. crash sites with multiple patients.
   B. incidents involving the rescue of a patient.
   C. shootings or stabbings of patients.
   D. patients who are intoxicated or have behavioral disorders.

3. While on the scene of an automobile crash, you find a power line of small diameter lying across the vehicle. You should:
   A. safely remove the power line by using rubber gloves and a long pipe or pole.
   B. wait for a power company worker to clear the scene prior to entering it because all power lines should be considered energized.
   C. enter the scene because power lines that are knocked down on the ground are grounded and pose no threat.
   D. remove the power line from the vehicle because power lines of small diameter are low energy and can be safely removed without injuring you.

4. During the scene size-up, you identify a hostile environment. You should:
   A. approach the scene cautiously to identify the number of patients.
   B. try to make brief contact with the patient to explain that you will return.
   C. retreat from the scene until law enforcement has controlled it.
   D. attempt to enter the scene and treat the patient as quickly as possible.

5. On a cold winter morning, you respond to a residence where several people are complaining of flu-like symptoms. Upon your arrival, you find the youngest child in the family to be unresponsive. You note no unusual odors in the house. You would suspect the patients could be suffering from:
   A. toxic inhalation.
   B. the influenza virus.
   C. hypothermia.
   D. food poisoning.

6. Which of the following scenes would most likely pose a threat to the EMT?
   A. a known crime scene
   B. a large crowd
   C. a hypoxic patient
   D. a bar with intoxicated patrons

7. Your major responsibility at a crime scene is to:
   A. provide emergency medical care.
   B. prevent unnecessary people from entering the scene.
   C. identify potential weapons and preserve evidence.
   D. console the family.

8. Immediately upon arriving at a vehicle crash scene, you should:
   A. identify the total number of patients.
   B. determine whether downed wires are present.
   C. assess the entire scene, looking for potential hazards.
   D. look for patients with life-threatening injuries.

9. A patient who opens his eyes when spoken to is documented as:
   A. disoriented, but responsive to verbal stimuli.
   B. responsive to verbal stimuli.
   C. alert but disoriented to person, place, and time.
   D. alert and oriented times three.

10. During the scene size-up and primary assessment, each call is typically categorized as being:
    A. a critical or noncritical call.
    B. due to a medical illness or traumatic injury.
    C. due to a traumatic injury or cardiac emergency.
    D. a cardiac emergency or respiratory distress.

11. In which patient would you try to determine the mechanism of injury?
    A. A patient who has a history of asthma and is wheezing.
    B. An unresponsive patient found on the street corner.
    C. A drug overdose patient who admits to taking multiple types of drugs.
    D. An elderly nursing home patient with blood in his stool.

12. Upon arrival on the scene, you determine that there are more patients than you and your partner can effectively provide emergency care for. When should you call for additional assistance?
    A. immediately after making the determination
    B. after conducting an primary assessment on each patient
    C. following a rapid trauma assessment of the two most critical patients
    D. after providing emergency care for each of the patients

13. You would determine the total number of patients at a scene during your:
    A. primary assessment.
    B. focused history and physical exam.
    C. rapid trauma assessment.
    D. scene size-up.

14. You arrive on the scene of a motor vehicle crash involving two cars and find four injured patients. The two patients who have been ejected from one of the vehicles appear to be severely injured. You should immediately:
    A. exit the ambulance and try to determine the most severely injured patient.
    B. identify the most critical patient, begin transport, and call for additional ambulances.
    C. immediately contact the hospital and ask it to prepare for four trauma patients.
    D. contact dispatch and request more ambulances to respond to the scene.

15. What two factors are used to categorize a patient as a trauma patient?
    A. scene size-up and the patient's vital signs
    B. immediate assessment of the scene and the primary patient assessment
    C. assessment of the scene and the mechanism of the patient's injury
    D. immediate assessment of the scene and the patient's mental status

16. While performing painful (tactile) stimulation to assess mental status, the patient responds with nonpurposeful movement. Which of the following is an example of nonpurposeful movement?

   A. The patient arches his back and flexes the arms towards the chest.

   B. The patient reaches up and grabs your hand in an attempt to remove pain.

   C. The patient makes attempts to move away from the painful stimulation.

   D. The patient moves his arm upward and outward in a sweeping motion toward the pain.

17. Which of the following is a sign of a partially occluded airway?

   A. a patient who has garbled speech

   B. an alert patient who has stridor on inhalation and is unable to speak

   C. a child who is crying vigorously and swallowing air

   D. an infant who is alert, sitting still, and drooling

18. You find a patient who is not alert lying supine on the floor at the bottom of the basement stairs. Your first priority should be to:

   A. determine the mental status.

   B. provide manual in-line spinal stabilization.

   C. open the airway using a head-tilt, chin-lift manuever.

   D. assess the radial pulse and skin temperature, color, and condition.

19. The most effective method to determine whether the depth of breathing is adequate is to:

   A. auscultate for breath sounds.

   B. inspect for retractions.

   C. apply a pulse oximeter.

   D. look, listen, and feel for air exchange.

20. During your primary assessment of an elderly patient found lying supine in bed at a nursing home, you determine that the patient is apneic. Your primary management should be to:

   A. immediately provide positive pressure ventilation.

   B. manually stabilize the cervical and lumbar spine.

   C. assess the circulation by checking a radial pulse.

   D. assess perfusion by checking the skin temperature.

21. You have been dispatched to the scene of a shooting. The local police have secured the scene and direct you to the patient who is a male about 16 years of age. There is a large bloodstain on the patient's left lateral chest region. The patient's eyes are closed and he does not move as you approach. Your partner takes manual in-line stabilization and opens the airway using the jaw-thrust maneuver. Your next immediate action should be to:

   A. apply a gauze dressing to the chest wound.

   B. assess the breathing status.

   C. size and place a cervical collar on the patient.

   D. palpate the chest for signs of chest injury.

22. You are providing positive pressure ventilation by bag-valve-mask device with an oropharyngeal airway in place. Your partner has sealed a sucking chest wound and controlled bleeding from the chest. You find that it is becoming increasingly difficult to squeeze the bag-valve-mask device to ventilate the patient. You should immediately:

   A. auscultate the chest for wheezing.

   B. recheck the patient's blood pressure.

   C. assess the breath sounds and neck.

   D. recheck the liter flow of oxygen to the bag-valve-mask device.

23. During your rapid trauma assessment, you find a bullet wound in the occipital region of the patient's head. The patient is unresponsive and his pupils are unequal in size. You should:
    A. quickly remove the oropharyngeal airway.
    B. decrease the oxygen concentration provided.
    C. ventilate the patient between 8 to 12 ventilations per minute.
    D. hyperventilate the patient at 20 ventilations per minute.

24. During the primary assessment, you are unable to ventilate an unresponsive infant. You have already repositioned the airway twice. Your next action should be to perform:
    A. five quick chest thrusts.
    B. five abdominal thrusts.
    C. a blind finger sweep.
    D. five rapid back blows.

25. The presence of a palpable radial pulse:
    A. indicates an estimated blood pressure at 100 mmHg diastolic.
    B. is not an accurate way to determine blood pressure.
    C. estimates the systolic blood pressure at 80 mmHg.
    D. provides an estimate of a diastolic blood pressure.

26. When initially assessing the pulse in a conscious adult, palpate the _____ artery, whereas in an infant you palpate the _____ artery.
    A. carotid, brachial
    B. radial, brachial
    C. radial, femoral
    D. brachial, radial

27. You arrive on the scene and find a patient who fell from a tree. His left pant leg is soaked with blood. You expose the injured area and find a large laceration with a steady flow of blood. You should immediately:
    A. press your gloved hand firmly over the wound.
    B. apply a tourniquet directly above the wound.
    C. place a pressure dressing over the wound site.
    D. apply digital pressure to the nearest proximal pressure point.

28. Which of the following skin temperature findings likely indicates that the patient has lost a significant amount of blood?
    A. hot
    B. warm
    C. cold
    D. cool

29. Capillary refill is a most reliable sign in:
    A. adults.
    B. elderly people.
    C. children less than six years of age.
    D. newborns.

30. When reconsidering the mechanism of injury in the secondary assessment, you should determine whether:
    A. the further evaluation of the mechanism of injury met criteria to be considered significant.
    B. any hazards or potential hazards that could harm you or the patient were missed.
    C. specific injury to organs can be identified.
    D. the airway or breathing is compromised.

31. Which of the following is *not* considered a significant mechanism of injury in the infant and child?
    A. falls of more than 10 feet.
    B. low-speed motor vehicle collisions.
    C. bicycle collisions.
    D. motor vehicle collision with the death of a passenger in the same compartment as the patient.

32. In what order would you assess a patient with a significant mechanism of injury?
    A. rapid trauma assessment, baseline vitals, SAMPLE history
    B. baseline vitals, rapid trauma assessment, SAMPLE history
    C. baseline vitals, SAMPLE history, rapid trauma assessment
    D. SAMPLE history, rapid trauma assessment, baseline vitals

33. You arrive at the scene of a motor vehicle crash that has significant vehicle damage. You find the patient unrestrained in the front seat. Following the scene size-up, you should immediately:
    A. perform an primary assessment.
    B. perform a focused physical exam to the head, chest, and abdomen.
    C. obtain a set of baseline vital signs.
    D. perform a rapid trauma assessment.

34. The rapid trauma assessment:
    A. focuses on a specific injury site.
    B. is a quick head-to-toe exam.
    C. begins with obtaining a SAMPLE history.
    D. does not include an assessment of vital signs.

35. The decision to perform a rapid trauma assessment or focused physical exam is based on the:
    A. baseline vital signs.
    B. SAMPLE history.
    C. mechanism of injury and primary assessment findings.
    D. findings in the ongoing assessment.

36. You performed a focused physical exam on a patient who suffered an isolated leg injury when his leg was caught in a piece of machinery. En route, the patient becomes disoriented and repeatedly asks you what happened. You should:
    A. contact medical direction for orders for additional emergency care.
    B. conduct a focused exam to the patient's head.
    C. obtain a SAMPLE history.
    D. perform a rapid trauma assessment.

37. A physical exam that is conducted to identify life-threatening injuries to the head, neck, chest, abdomen, pelvis, extremities, and posterior body is:
    A. a focused trauma exam.
    B. an ongoing assessment.
    C. an primary assessment.
    D. a rapid trauma assessment.

38. You find the patient complaining of severe pain to his ankle following a fall while playing basketball. When questioned, he cannot identify where he is. You should perform:
    A. a rapid medical assessment.
    B. a focused physical exam.
    C. a rapid trauma assessment.
    D. an primary assessment and rapid transport.

39. The mnemonic DCAP-BTLS stands for:
    A. deformities, contusions, avulsions, pooling blood, breaks, trauma, lacerations, swelling.
    B. deformities, contusions, avulsions, penetrations, breaks, tenderness, lacerations, swelling.
    C. deformities, contusions, abrasions, punctures, burns, tenderness, lacerations, swelling.
    D. distention, contusions, abrasions, punctures, burns, tenderness, lacerations, swelling.

40. The rapid trauma assessment is best described as:
    A. a focused exam of specific injury sites to the patient.
    B. a physical exam to identify all injuries to the patient.
    C. an exam to identify potential life-threatening injuries to the patient.
    D. a reassessment of the components of the primary assessment.

41. When assessing the head and face of a trauma patient during the secondary assessment, you should:
    A. remove the head immobilization device to allow for a better examination of the head.
    B. firmly press on the skull, using the tips of your fingers to feel for depressions.
    C. note any areas of tenderness or swelling to the maxilla and mandible.
    D. apply pressure to each eye, assessing for injury to the globe.

42. While assessing the chest during the rapid trauma secondary assessment, you find minimal chest rise during inhalation. You should:
    A. complete the assessment followed by applying oxygen by nonrebreather mask.
    B. complete the assessment and then provide positive pressure ventilation.
    C. immediately administer oxygen by nonrebreather mask and then continue the assessment.
    D. immediately begin positive pressure ventilation and continue the assessment.

43. When performing a rapid trauma assessment, which of the following represents a critical finding that must be managed immediately?
    A. paradoxical chest wall movement
    B. a closed fibia fracture
    C. flat jugular veins with patient sitting at a 45°
    D. an open humerus fracture with the bone protruding from the skin

44. The rapid trauma assessment is performed to:
    A. obtain a set of baseline vital signs.
    B. identify life-threatening injuries or conditions.
    C. identify and manage life threats to the airway and ventilation.
    D. identify detailed information about the injury.

45. When assessing a medical patient, it is important to ask questions concerning the chief complaint to:
    A. further assess the history of the present illness.
    B. formulate your complete plan of treatment.
    C. determine whether advanced life support (ALS) assistance is needed.
    D. determine the mechanism of injury.

46. Which mnemonic is used to collect information about the chief complaint?
    A. A and O × 3
    B. DCAP-BTLS
    C. AVPU
    D. OPQRST

47. The mnemonic OPQRST is used to assess:
    A. onset, pain, quantity, radiation, sensation, time.
    B. onset, provocation/palliation, quality, radiation, severity, time.
    C. onset, pain, quality, radiation, sensation, time.
    D. onset, provocation, quantity, radiation, sensation, time.

48. When asking the patient about provocation/palliation, you are trying to determine:
    A. what makes the symptom better or worse.
    B. what started the symptom.
    C. the approximate time the symptom started.
    D. what the patient was doing when the symptoms were first noticed.

49. While assessing a patient's complaint, you ask, "Does the pain move to the jaw or down the arms?" This question is assessing the:
    A. quality.
    B. radiation.
    C. provocation.
    D. severity.

50. When assessing the *quality* of a patient's chest pain, you would ask:
    A. What does the pain feel like?
    B. Where is the pain?
    C. What makes the pain worse?
    D. When and how did the pain begin?

51. The history and physical during the secondary assessment for the responsive medical patient is performed in what sequence?
    A. history, focused physical exam, vital signs
    B. history, vital signs, focused physical exam
    C. focused physical exam, vital signs, history
    D. vital signs, history, focused physical exam

52. Assessment of the unresponsive medical patient is performed in which sequence?
    A. history, rapid medical assessment, vital signs
    B. history, vital signs, rapid medical assessment
    C. rapid medical assessment, vital signs, history
    D. vital signs, history, rapid medical assessment

53. An unresponsive medical patient is:
    A. a low priority.
    B. a medium priority.
    C. a high priority.
    D. not a priority because he is a medical patient.

54. When assessing the unresponsive medical patient:
    A. perform a complete detailed secondary assessment prior to transport.
    B. inspect the scene for information about the nature of the illness.
    C. do not ask bystanders and family members questions regarding the incident.
    D. perform the primary assessment after the rapid medical assessment.

55. Unequal pupils can indicate:
    A. carbon monoxide poisoning.
    B. head injury.
    C. severe hypoxia.
    D. heat emergency.

56. Your medical patient responds to painful (tactile) stimuli with nonpurposeful movement during the primary assessment. After the primary assessment, you should next perform a:
    A. focused physical exam.
    B. SAMPLE history.
    C. detailed physical assessment of the head.
    D. rapid medical assessment.

57. The unresponsive medical patient should be placed in which position?
    A. Trendelenburg position
    B. semi-Fowler position
    C. prone position, legs extended
    D. lateral recumbent position

58. You have just completed the primary assessment of a medical patient complaining of shortness of breath. You would next:
    A. perform a rapid medical secondary assessment.
    B. evaluate the chief complaint using the OPQRST mnemonic.
    C. perform certain components of a detailed physical exam.
    D. perform a focused exam of the chest.

59. The purpose of a detailed secondary assessment is to:
    A. identify and manage all nonlife-threatening injuries.
    B. identify all life-threatening injuries and manage those injuries.
    C. reevaluate the primary assessment and assess all interventions.
    D. determine whether the mechanism of injury correlates with the patient's injuries.

60. You have just loaded a trauma patient with multiple injuries into the ambulance for transport. The next assessment to be performed is:
    A. an primary assessment.
    B. a rapid trauma assessment.
    C. a detailed secondary assessment.
    D. an ongoing assessment.

61. Which component would be assessed during the detailed secondary assessment only, not during the rapid trauma assessment?
    A. inspection of the conjunctiva
    B. evaluation of breath sounds
    C. palpation of the abdomen
    D. assessment of pupillary function

62. What condition would you suspect if you found yellow sclera during your assessment?
    A. congestive heart failure
    B. liver failure
    C. narcotic drug overdose
    D. head injury

63. A trauma patient presents with a swollen neck and crepitation upon palpation. You would most likely suspect trauma to the:
    A. head.
    B. trachea.
    C. abdomen.
    D. spine.

64. During the assessment of a patient who fell, you find a portion of the chest wall that moves inward during inspiration and then moves outward during exhalation. The condition the patient is suffering is a:
    A. flail chest.
    B. tension pneumothorax.

C. simple pneumothorax.

D. collapsed lung.

65. Injuries found during the secondary assessment are managed:

A. after the completion of the exam.

B. when found during the exam.

C. after the patient is transported.

D. just prior to patient transport.

66. A trauma patient is unable to close his mouth. Your major concern is:

A. maintenance of spinal immobilization.

B. potential damage to teeth.

C. immobilizing a fracture of the maxilla.

D. maintaining a patent airway.

67. When examining the eyes of a patient during the secondary assessment:

A. it is necessary to remove any foreign bodies embedded in the eye to further examine it.

B. the eyelid should be forced open if injuries to the eyelid are observed.

C. both pupils should react simultaneously to a light shone in one eye.

D. pressure should be applied to the globe of the eye to control bleeding.

68. A pupil that is large in size and not responding to light is referred to as:

A. profiled.

B. fixed and dilated.

C. pytosis.

D. false dilation.

69. The eyes moving together in one direction is referred to as:

A. visual acuity.

B. consensual movement.

C. conjugate movement.

D. conjugate gaze.

70. An alert and oriented patient presents with one pupil that is fixed and dilated. You should suspect a:

A. severe head injury with brain herniation.

B. stroke with bleeding inside the cranium.

C. concussion from a blow to the head.

D. possible direct injury to the eye.

71. During palpation of a trauma patient's neck, you feel an unusual sensation of air under the skin. This is referred to as:

A. a tension pneumothorax.

B. a pericardial tamponade.

C. hematoma infiltration.

D. subcutaneous emphysema.

72. Pale oral mucous membranes can indicate:

A. severe hypoxia.

B. infection.

C. acute blood loss from an injury.

D. blood loss over a long period of time.

73. Wheezing upon auscultation of the chest usually indicates:

A. fluid in the terminal air sacs and alveoli.

B. decreased airway resistance in the smaller bronchioles.

C. constricton of the trachea and bronchi.

D. constriction and inflammation of the bronchiole.

74. A purpose of conducting an ongoing assessment is to:

A. determine whether the patient's condition has worsened or imporved.

B. make sure you did not miss any life-threatening injuries in the rapid trauma exam.

C. perform a more detailed examination of the head.

D. identify all other nonlife-threatening injuries and manage them as they are found.

75. You respond to a scene to find a patient who was struck on the head with a hammer. The family indicates that he lost consciousness for approximately 5 minutes prior to your arrival. The patient is disoriented. The ongoing assessment should be repeated every:
    A. 3 minutes.
    B. 5 minutes.
    C. 10 minutes.
    D. 15 minutes.

76. You are managing a patient who called EMS after he fainted. En route to the hospital, the patient begins to experience a sharp tearing pain that radiates to his lower back. You should immediately:
    A. do a rapid medical assessment to identify life threats.
    B. do a detailed exam of the abdomen and report the results to medical direction.
    C. repeat the SAMPLE history to be sure you did not miss anything.
    D. perform an ongoing assessment to include a focused exam of the abdomen.

77. You are called to the scene for an unresponsive 76-year-old female patient who is suspected of having had a stroke. You open the patient's airway with a head-tilt, chin-lift maneuver. Your partner informs you that the respiratory rate is 22 per minute. You should immediately:
    A. assess the radial pulse.
    B. begin bag-valve-mask ventilation.
    C. perform a rapid medical assessment.
    D. assess the depth of the respirations.

78. The primary purpose for taking several sets of vital signs in a patient is to:
    A. be sure that the previous sets of vital signs were accurate.
    B. meet the requirements of the protocol that you are functioning under when treating patients.
    C. make the patient feel more comfortable by having him think you are performing more treatment.
    D. identify trends in the patient's condition that could indicate improvement or deterioration.

79. You are treating a 26-year-old patient who dropped a brick on his foot at a construction site. His foot is deformed, swollen, and painful. The patient denies having fallen to the ground and is found seated in a chair on your arrival. He complains that "my foot is killing me." His respirations are 20 per minute with full depth, and his radial pulse is 102 per minute. His skin is warm, dry, and a normal color. You should next:
    A. repeat the primary assessment.
    B. do a rapid trauma assessment.
    C. perform a focused physical exam of the injured foot.
    D. conduct an ongoing assessment and get a set of vital signs.

80. You are en route to the hospital with a 34-year-old female patient who was involved in a motor vehicle crash. After reconnecting the nonrebreather supply tubing to the on-board oxygen flow meter, you note that the patient no longer has her eyes open. You should immediately:
    A. assess the carotid pulse.
    B. ask the patient to open her eyes.

C. begin bag-valve-mask ventilation.

D. open the airway with a jaw thrust manuever.

81. During the ongoing assessment of a patient involved in a bar fight, you note that his pulse rate has decreased severely and has become weak. You should suspect:

A. a low blood sugar level (hypoglycemia).

B. a head injury.

C. a heat-related emergency.

D. an allergic reaction (anaphylaxis).

82. Which of the following would cause you to repeat an ongoing assessment every 5 minutes?

A. a respiratory rate of 24 per minute

B. equal pupils that constrict to light

C. an isolated fracture of the radius and ulna

D. a laceration of the hand with oozing blood

83. Why should you wait at least 1 second after you push the transmit button before you begin speaking into the radio microphone?

A. to eliminate static in the background

B. to help your battery last longer

C. to allow the radio to broadcast farther

D. to allow the repeater time to open the channel and prevent cutting off the first part of the communication

84. After you are finished with your radio transmission, you should:

A. turn the radio off to save power.

B. say "Over" and wait for confirmation from the other participant.

C. say "Over" and turn your radio off to free the airwaves.

D. wait 2 seconds and ask for confirmation of your communication.

85. Identify the correct sequence for communicating patient information to medical direction.

1. patient age and sex
2. history of present illness
3. chief complaint
4. past illness
5. vitals
6. mental status

A. 1, 2, 3, 5, 6, 4

B. 1, 3, 2, 6, 5, 4

C. 1, 3, 2, 4, 6, 5

D. 1, 3, 5, 6, 2, 4

86. Once you have received a correct order from medical direction, you should:

A. repeat the order back word for word.

B. ask medical direction to repeat the order.

C. repeat the order to dispatch.

D. ask your partner to repeat the order to you.

87. Clear communication with medical direction is most important because:

A. patient confidentiality statutes must be followed.

B. the Federal Communications Commission requires accurate transmission of information.

C. medical legal liability is a primary concern.

D. receiving accurate orders is necessary for good patient care.

88. Essential information that needs to be summarized in the oral report includes the:
    A. patient's chief complaint, vital signs at the scene, treatment given en route, response to the treatment, and pertinent history not given earlier.
    B. patient's chief complaint, vital signs en route, and treatment en route.
    C. patient's chief complaint, vital signs taken en route, treatment given en route, response to the treatment, and pertinent history not given earlier.
    D. patient's chief complaint, vital signs en route, and treatment given.

89. To improve communication with your patient, especially children and infants, you should:
    A. immediately establish that you are in charge and allow the patient to speak only to you.
    B. position yourself at the same level or lower than that of the patient.
    C. address all patients by their first name.
    D. remove any family, toys, or other distracters from the area directly around the patient.

90. You are assessing an 84-year-old male patient. When you ask him a question, there is a long delay before he answers. You should:
    A. face the patient and speak much more loudly.
    B. ask the patient to respond more quickly to the questions.
    C. allow enough time for the patient to respond to your questions.
    D. start asking the family or relatives at the scene the questions instead of the patient.

91. Information given in the oral report:
    A. is not important because a written report is always provided.
    B. is important because it helps the hospital ensure continuity of care.
    C. generally requires only your unit identification and the patient's chief complaint.
    D. is of little importance because the hospital staff will make their own assessment.

92. Which of the following is an appropriate procedure when using the radio to communicate with other members of the EMS team?
    A. Push the press to talk (PTT) button and immediately begin speaking.
    B. Speak with your mouth at least 12 to 18 inches from the microphone.
    C. Give objective or relevant subjective information and avoid offering a diagnosis.
    D. After receiving medical control orders, stop the transmission and initiate treatment.

93. The agency responsible for licensing radio base stations is the:
    A. Health Insurance Portability and Accountability Act.
    B. Federal Communications Commission.
    C. Department of Transportation.
    D. National Highway Traffic Safety Administration.

94. A major disadvantage of the use of cellular telephones in EMS is that they:
    A. require a special EMS license from the Federal Communications Commission.
    B. do not work well in urban areas.
    C. can be overwhelmed in a disaster.
    D. are expensive to maintain and operate.

95. A device that receives a transmission from a relatively low-powered source such as a mobile radio and rebroadcasts the signal on another frequency and a higher power is called a(n):
    A. encoder.
    B. duplexer.
    C. repeater.
    D. decoder.

96. When used in Emergency Medical Service dispatching, CAD stands for:
    A. computer-aided dispatch.
    B. critical-area dispatch.
    C. common-area dispatch.
    D. constant-action dispatch.

97. Response times as stated by the emergency medical dispatcher:
    A. should be accurately transcribed to the EMS report by the EMT.
    B. do not need to be precisely recorded by the EMT.
    C. are not required in EMS systems.
    D. are generally handled only by the Emergency Medical Dispatcher.

98. The agency that has jurisdiction over all EMS radio operations in the United States is the:
    A. Department of Health and Human Services.
    B. National Highway Traffic Safety Administration.
    C. Department of Transportation.
    D. Federal Communications Commission.

99. If you believe that you have received an inappropriate order from medical direction, you should:
    A. perform the order and not question medical direction.
    B. question medical direction about the order prior to continuing.
    C. perform the order and document the order on the EMS report.
    D. contact your supervisor for further instructions.

100. Medical direction insists that you perform a procedure outside your scope of practice. You should:
    A. question the order, perform the procedure if medical direction continues to insist that you do so, and document your reason for doing it on the EMS report form.
    B. not question the medical direction authority and perform the order.
    C. contact your supervisor to respond to the scene prior to performing the order from medical direction.
    D. disregard the order, continue with patient care, and document the incident thoroughly on a special incident report form after the call.

101. When speaking to an elderly patient who has been in a vehicle crash, you should:
    A. speak loudly and assertively with authority.
    B. use medical terms to convey intelligence.
    C. speak slowly, calmly, and distinctly.
    D. use codes to protect the patient from stress.

102. The patient care report must include:
    A. chief complaint, level of responsiveness, and blood pressure.
    B. skin color, temperature, and condition.
    C. pulse rate, respiratory rate, and effort.
    D. all of the above.

103. After communicating your arrival on the scene, according to the Department of Transportation, the next communication should be:
    A. your arrival at the hospital.
    B. when you leave the scene and are en route to the hospital.
    C. when you arrive at the patient's side.
    D. when you transfer the care of the patient to the hospital staff.

104. The Department of Transportation requires minimum data to be collected on the prehospital care report (PCR). Which is an element of the Department of Transportation's minimum data set?
    A. patient's legal name
    B. patient's level of responsiveness
    C. patient's age and sex
    D. patient's diastolic blood pressure

105. The narrative section of the patient care report (PCR) should include the patient's:
    A. chief complaint.
    B. name.
    C. sex.
    D. systolic blood pressure.

106. What is an acceptable abbreviation for "four times a day"?
    A. QID
    B. SOB
    C. TID
    D. NTG

107. Information that the Department of Transportation requires on all patient care reports is called the:
    A. transport care information.
    B. DOT PCR data.
    C. minimum data set.
    D. DOT patient care information.

108. An important consideration related to the collection of information for patient care reports is that:
    A. clocks do not need to be accurate and synchronous.
    B. only one set of vital signs needs to be recorded to limit the use of space.
    C. the diagnosis of the patient's condition is reported in the narrative section.
    D. the patient's information can be shared with any health care provider.

109. Documenting signs or symptoms that were not found during the assessment would be referred to as a:
    A. pertinent negative.
    B. negative complaint.
    C. reverse symptom.
    D. compound complaint.

110. Knowingly providing false information on the patient care report:
    A. is acceptable if limited to only the vital signs.
    B. is acceptable if an act of omission occurs.
    C. is acceptable if an act of commission occurs.
    D. is never acceptable.

111. Patient refusals of treatment require:
    A. less documentation than for a transported patient.
    B. about the same amount of information as a transported patient.
    C. complete documentation of your efforts to provide care.
    D. more documentation than for a transported patient.

112. Keeping the information contained in the patient care report confidential is:
    A. the responsibility of the information officer.
    B. necessary only if required by local or state law.

C. required only if the patient makes a formal request.

D. your responsibility as a field EMS provider.

113. If a patient refuses to sign your refusal document, you should:

    A. leave the scene before the patient changes his mind.

    B. place an X in the refusal box.

    C. restrain the patient, perform an assessment, treat the patient, and transport him if he continues to refuse to sign.

    D. have a family member, police officer, or bystander sign the report verifying that the patient refused to sign.

114. When a patient signs a refusal, the EMT must be completely sure that the patient:

    A. will not sue the EMT.

    B. will be able to call 911 if his condition deteriorates later.

    C. does not have a significant past medical history.

    D. is competent and able to make a rational decision about his care.

115. In the refusal report, the EMT should include all of the following information *except:*

    A. a complete patient assessment or documentation explaining why it was not completed.

    B. a statement that the EMT advised the patient of the consequences of refusing transport, including the potential of death.

    C. a statement advising the patient not to call EMS if the patient will not allow the EMT to perform his job.

    D. the documentation of any and all communication with medical direction or other authorities.

116. To correct an error in the patient care report (PCR), you should:

    A. erase the error completely; then write over the area with the correction.

    B. draw a single horizontal line through the error; then initial the correction.

    C. write directly over the error with a different color ink; then initial the correction.

    D. cover the error completely with correction fluid; then write directly over the area.

Scenario

Questions 117–119 refer to the following scenario:

You and your partner Emil are dispatched to the scene of a fight at 69 Over Street. Dispatch advises that the police have secured the scene and request you to expedite your response. Upon your arrival, you are met by a police officer who states that an elderly man named Carl Luis has been shot in the chest. As you approach the patient, you quickly gain the impression that he is severely injured. You see blood escaping freely from a penetrating wound to the upper right chest. The patient is breathing approximately 20 times a minute.

117. As you proceed with the primary assessment, your first action should be to:

    A. assess mental status using the mnemonic AVPU.

    B. assess airway, breathing, and circulation.

    C. perform a focused physical exam of the chest.

    D. place your gloved hand over the chest wound.

118. The next action performed as part of the primary assessment of this patient is to:
    A. open the airway using the head-tilt, chin-lift maneuver.
    B. assess mental status using the mnemonic AVPU.
    C. obtain a SAMPLE history and a detailed exam.
    D. establish manual in-line stabilization of the spine.

119. In relation to this patient's mechanism of injury, which types of physical exam should you perform?
    A. focused trauma assessment
    B. rapid trauma assessment
    C. detailed physical assessment
    D. concentrated trauma assessment

120. You have responded to a call for a patient who fell. You arrive on scene and find the patient with a deformity to the toe. The patient requests care and transport. The hospital is located close by. Your departmental policy requires at least two sets of vital signs to be taken on all patients. Due to your close proximity to the hospital, you obtain only one set. How should you handle this situation?
    A. Report the same vital signs as recorded earlier.
    B. Use a standard set of vitals based on the age.
    C. Document that you failed to obtain the vital signs.
    D. Use the same vital signs but change them slightly.

121. While completing your patient care report, you note that the patient complained of intense pain in his toe. This is an example of _____ information.
    A. subjective
    B. orthopedic
    C. minor
    D. objective

122. You are returning to the station and stop at a convenience store to purchase a soft drink. A gentleman approaches and asks what was going on across the street from his house a few minutes ago. He identifies himself as the neighbor of the patient you just transported. How do you respond to his request?
    A. Tell him exactly what happened but do not use any names.
    B. Tell him only if he promises not to tell where he got the information.
    C. Tell him this is off the record and then relay the information.
    D. Tell him you are not allowed to divulge such information.

123. You arrive on the scene and find a 27-year-old man in the bathroom of his home. During your primary assessment, you determine that he is not alert. The next immediate action you should take is to:
    A. open his airway by using a jaw-thrust maneuver.
    B. ask him to open his eyes or talk to you.
    C. insert an oropharyngeal airway.
    D. check for a radial pulse and skin color, temperature, and condition.

124. You arrive on the scene and find a young male construction worker who was crushed under a wall that collapsed on top of him. You determine that the scene is safe and approach the patient. He is severely cyanotic and appears not to be breathing. Blood is spurting out of his cut pant leg. Your next immediate action is to:
    A. begin positive pressure ventilation with supplemental oxygen.
    B. expose and apply direct pressure to the bleeding leg wound.
    C. assess the radial pulse and skin for perfusion status.
    D. take manual in-line stabilization and apply a nonrebreather mask.

125. You arrive on the scene and find a 30-year-old male patient with a gunshot wound to the chest. While conducting your general impression, you note blood in the mouth, severe cyanosis to the face and neck, and no chest wall movement. You should immediately:
    A. suction the airway and occlude the gunshot wound to the chest.
    B. expose the patient and check for other serious gunshot wounds.
    C. begin bag-value-mask ventilation with supplemental oxygen and place your gloved hand over the wound.
    D. occlude the open wound, apply a nonrebreather mask at 15 lpm, and begin your primary assessment.

126. You are assessing a 40-year-old male patient who crashed his motorcycle. He complains of pain to his right leg. You suspect that the tibia and fibula are fractured. Which of the following would be the best indicator of a suspected fracture?
    A. crepitation
    B. pain
    C. ecchymosis
    D. edema

127. Which of the following provides the *least* accurate information about the perfusion status when you are assessing circulation in the adult patient?
    A. capillary refill
    B. skin color
    C. skin condition
    D. peripheral pulse

128. While conducting your general impression, which of the following would cause you to believe the patient is dyspneic?
    A. The patient is gasping for air while crying loudly.
    B. The patient is lying supine on the couch while explaining how he feels.

C. The patient says a few words and takes a breath.
    D. The patient is on home oxygen at 2 lpm.

129. You arrive on the scene of an auto crash and find a 23-year-old woman who was the driver of the vehicle. During the primary assessment, you find cyanosis to her face and neck, a large depression with moderate bleeding to her left temporal region, a respiratory rate of 12 per minute with shallow breathing, and weak peripheral pulses. You should immediately:
    A. apply direct pressure to the head injury and apply a nonrebreather mask at 15 lpm.
    B. perform a jaw-thrust maneuver and begin positive pressure ventilation with supplemental oxygen.
    C. take a blood pressure and apply a pulse oximeter to determine the blood oxygen concentration.
    D. dress the wound to the head and then begin bag-valve-mask ventilation with supplemental oxygen.

130. A 25-year-old female patient was thrown off her horse. She is responsive and complains of pain to her head. Following the primary assessment you should:
    A. conduct a focused physical exam of the head.
    B. begin transport.
    C. conduct a detailed exam of the head.
    D. conduct a rapid trauma assessment.

131. You arrive on the scene and find a 28-year-old female who fell 20 feet while roofing a house. As you exit the ambulance, she appears to be unresponsive. You notice a large pool of blood around her left thigh. Blood is draining from the mouth and nose. Your first priority is to:

    A. suction the airway and begin bag-valve-mask ventilation.

    B. look for safety hazards before approaching the patient.

    C. expose the left thigh and find any possible major bleeding.

    D. open her airway using a jaw-thrust maneuver and apply a nonrebreather mask at 15 lpm.

132. You arrive on the scene and find a 10-year-old male patient who was struck by a car while riding his bike. He is unresponsive to painful stimuli. You have opened the airway with a jaw-thrust maneuver and find the respirations to be 24 per minute and shallow. His radial pulse is barely palpable. You should immediately:

    A. apply a nonrebreather mask at 15 lpm.

    B. begin chest compressions.

    C. begin bag-valve-mask ventilation.

    D. apply a cervical spinal immobilization collar.

133. A 62-year-old female patient whom you find sitting in her recliner at home is complaining of severe abdominal pain as you walk in the door. As you approach the patient, she states that her "belly is real sore and aching bad." Your next action in assessing the patient is to:

    A. assess the circulation and gather a SAMPLE history.

    B. open the airway and assess the breathing status.

    C. begin bag-valve-mask ventilation and connect supplemental oxygen.

    D. conduct a rapid medical assessment and assess vital signs.

134. You arrive on the scene and find an eight-year-old boy at the local gym who was knocked out while playing basketball. Following your assessment, you suspect that he has a head injury. You should immediately:

    A. transport without treatment because of the lack of parental consent.

    B. initiate emergency care and transport.

    C. wait for the police to arrive before initiating treatment.

    D. contact the parents for consent to begin treatment.

135. You arrive on the scene and find a 23-year-old female patient who stepped on a piece of glass and lacerated her foot while walking through the front yard. She is sitting on the ground holding her foot as you approach her. She complains that her foot "hurts really bad" and is bleeding. Your next immediate action is to:

    A. assess the amount of bleeding to determine whether it is uncontrolled and major.

    B. apply a nonrebreather mask at 15 lpm.

    C. immediately begin a rapid trauma assessment to assess for life-threatening injuries.

    D. perform a jaw-thrust maneuver and assess the breathing status.

136. Following the primary assessment of a medical patient complaining of chest pain, you determine that he is not oriented and is speaking inappropriately. The next step in your assessment is to:

    A. repeat the primary assessment.

    B. perform an ongoing assessment.

    C. conduct a focused physical exam of the chest.

    D. perform a rapid medical assessment.

137. You arrive on the scene of an auto crash involving a frontal collision and find the patient seated in the front seat on the driver's side of the vehicle. You determine that the scene is safe and approach the patient. You should immediately:
    A. determine the patient's mental status.
    B. open the patient's airway using the jaw-thrust maneuver.
    C. establish manual in-line stabilization of the patient's head and neck.
    D. assess the patient's radial pulse, carotid pulses, and skin.

138. Tracheal deviation is:
    A. an early sign of a pneumothorax.
    B. a late sign of a tension pneumothorax.
    C. a sign of pericardial tamponade.
    D. a late sign of hypovolemic shock.

139. You arrive on the scene and find a 20-year-old male patient who was involved in an auto crash. Upon your assessment, you note that he cannot tell you what date it is, where he is, or whom he is with. The patient refuses to let you examine him further and refuses any emergency care. You should:
    A. have the patient sign a refusal form and leave the scene.
    B. turn the patient over to the police on the scene and leave.
    C. begin to administer emergency care to the patient and then transport him, using restraints if necessary.
    D. have the police place the patient under protective custody so that you can administer emergency care.

140. Capillary refill is most reliable and provides the most information on which of the following patients?
    A. a three-year-old trauma patient who is trapped in a vehicle in 10°F temperature
    B. an eight-year-old who is having an asthma attack

C. a 30-year-old who was shot in the chest three times
    D. a five-year-old who lacerated his femoral artery on broken glass and is bleeding profusely

141. Blood mixed with clear fluid coming from the ears in a patient who was struck in the head would most likely indicate:
    A. a fractured skull.
    B. a concussion.
    C. an injury to the ear canal.
    D. a lacerated meningeal artery.

142. You arrive on the scene and find a 65-year-old male sitting on the couch at home complaining that he "can't breathe." The respiratory rate is 28 per minute with full chest rise. The SpO_2 is 88 percent. The patient is alert and oriented, and his radial pulse is rapid and strong. His skin is slightly pale, cool, and clammy. You should immediately:
    A. apply a nonrebreather mask at 15 lpm.
    B. assess his baseline vital signs.
    C. perform a rapid medical exam.
    D. place the patient in a supine position.

143. You arrive on the scene and find a 74-year-old male who collapsed at home. As you approach him, you note that his eyes are not open, you hear a loud gurgling noise, and it appears that he is breathing at about six times per minute. You should immediately:
    A. assess the radial and then the carotid pulse.
    B. begin bag-valve-mask ventilation with supplemental oxygen and assess his mental status.
    C. apply a nonrebreather mask and assess the blood pressure.
    D. suction the mouth until it is clear and then begin positive pressure ventilation.

144. The respiratory rate of an infant:
    A. is approximately the same as that of an adult.
    B. is usually slightly slower than that of an adult.
    C. is higher at birth and progressively decreases with age.
    D. is irregularly irregular.

145. Which of the following is the best indicator of hypoxia in a patient complaining of dyspnea?
    A. The patient states that his difficulty breathing is a ten on the severity scale.
    B. The pulse oximeter reads 93 percent while the patient is on a nonrebreather mask at 15 lpm.
    C. The skin is slightly pale, cool, and clammy.
    D. The patient is using his sternocleidomastoid muscles to breathe and you see intercostal retractions.

146. You arrive on the scene and find a patient who is complaining of dizziness and nausea. The respirations are 18 per minute with good tidal volume and the (SpO_2) reading is 96 percent. You find that the radial pulse is present and the skin is warm, moist, and flushed. You should next:
    A. determine the level of responsiveness.
    B. begin a rapid medical assessment.
    C. gather a SAMPLE history.
    D. assess the patient's abdomen for tenderness and rigidity.

147. The skin is assessed during the primary assessment to determine the patient's:
    A. level of hypoxia.
    B. number of circulating red blood cells.
    C. perfusion status.
    D. need for oxygen therapy.

148. Which of the following is considered a life-threatening injury?
    A. fractured ribs
    B. large laceration that is oozing blood
    C. open wound to the posterior thorax
    D. severely deformed humerus

Scenario

Questions 149 and 150 refer to the following scenario:

You arrive on the scene and find a 77-year-old male patient lying in bed. He does not respond to verbal stimuli. He is breathing at 22 times per minute with good tidal volume and his radial pulse is 78 per minute. His pulse oximetry (SpO_2) reading is 93 percent. The skin is warm, dry, and normal in color.

149. Your next immediate action for this patient is to:
    A. apply a nasal cannula at 2 lpm and begin a rapid medical assessment.
    B. establish manual in-line spinal stabilization and insert an oropharyngeal airway.
    C. obtain a set of baseline vital signs and begin transport.
    D. begin bag-valve-mask ventilation with supplemental oxygen.

150. The skin of the patient most likely indicates:
    A. hypovolemic shock.
    B. inadequate delivery of hemoglobin to the cells.
    C. good tissue perfusion.
    D. hypoxia and hypercarbia.

151. The unresponsive medical patient should be placed in what position?
    A. supine with head slightly elevated
    B. Fowler's
    C. left lateral recumbent
    D. Trendelenburg

152. Which of the following is considered subjective patient information?
    A. "The patient has a swollen, deformed extremity."
    B. "The patient's pulse is 110 beats per minute."
    C. "The patient's blood pressure was 110/80."
    D. "The patient is in pain."

Scenario

Questions 153 and 154 refer to the following scenario:

As you are pulling up to the scene of a construction accident, you spot a patient lying prone on the ground next to a pile of rubble. It appears that a building has collapsed.

153. Your first priority is to:
    A. establish in-line spinal stabilization and logroll the patient onto his back.
    B. assess the patient's mental status and determine whether he is responsive.
    C. search for more than one patient and call for additional resources.
    D. wait by the ambulance until the engineer has indicated that the structure is safe to enter.

154. The next step in managing the patient is to:
    A. roll the patient onto his side to check for responsiveness and an open airway.
    B. insert an oropharyngeal airway and begin positive pressure ventilation.
    C. establish manual in-line spinal stabilization and logroll the patient into a supine position.
    D. gather a SAMPLE history from someone at the scene while your partner takes a set of baseline vital signs.

155. A detailed physical exam is performed:
    A. to identify and manage life-threatening injuries.
    B. to identify and manage other nonlife-threatening injuries.
    C. to determine trends in the patient's condition.
    D. before any emergency care can be done.

156. Which of the following breath sounds are expected in a patient with alveoli that collapse after exhalation and re-expand with each inhalation?
    A. crackles (rales)
    B. wheezing
    C. pleural friction rub
    D. rhonchi

157. You arrive on the scene and find a 16-year-old male patient lying on the living room floor in a fetal position (curled up with his knees drawn to his chest). His positioning would cause you most likely to suspect he is suffering from:
    A. an asthma attack.
    B. congestive heart failure.
    C. appendicitis.
    D. a migraine.

158. When assessing the patient's pupils during the detailed physical exam, you shine the light in the right eye while inspecting the left pupil reaction. This is testing the:
    A. consensual reflex.
    B. extra ocular eye movements.
    C. muscle palsies.
    D. sclera.

159. You arrive on the scene of a bar fight and find an approximately 26-year-old male patient who was struck several times in the face. The patient is hostile and not cooperating. He cannot remember his address or his last name and does not know where he is. He refuses to allow you to assess him or provide any emergency care. You should:

    A. have him sign a refusal form and leave the scene.

    B. explain the consequences of not allowing you to assess and treat him, document it on the prehospital care report (PCR), and have the patient and a witness sign the refusal form.

    C. call for the police, restrain the patient, and conduct a secondary assessment to identify any life-threatening injuries.

    D. have his friend who is at the bar with him drive him to the hospital as you follow close behind.

160. You arrive on the scene and find a 23-year-old pregnant patient trapped in her car that is on its roof following a broadside collision. Upon arrival at the scene, you should:

    A. gain access to the vehicle and take manual in-line spinal stabilization.

    B. immediately apply a nonrebreather mask at 15 lpm to the patient to try to protect the fetus.

    C. contact a second ambulance in case the patient goes into labor and delivers at the scene.

    D. wait until the fire department has stabilized the vehicle before gaining access to the patient.

161. A 40-year-old male patient was struck in the face by a softball. During your detailed exam, you note that both of his eyes deviate upward with a conjugate gaze. You would suspect he is possibly suffering from:

    A. an infraorbital fracture.

    B. a nasal fracture.

    C. a zygomatic contusion.

    D. a third cranial nerve injury.

162. During your rapid trauma assessment of a patient who fell down the steps, you note that the unresponsive patient's left pupil is fixed and dilated. You would suspect that the patient most likely has:

    A. suffered a brain injury.

    B. injured the eighth cranial nerve.

    C. injured the eyeball during the fall.

    D. fractured the maxilla and mandible.

163. If the left pupil is fixed and dilated in a patient with a brain injury you would suspect that the impact and injury most likely occurred to which side of the head?

    A. frontal region

    B. left region

    C. right region

    D. occipital region

164. *Priapism* is the term for:

    A. a persistent erection of the penis.

    B. dissection of the abdominal aorta.

    C. air in the thoracic cavity.

    D. pelvic instability.

Scenario

Questions 165 and 166 refer to the following scenario:

You arrive on the scene and find a 34-year-old female patient who crashed her motorcycle. During your assessment, you note that her skin is pale, cool, and clammy, her abdomen is rigid and tender, and her radial pulse is weak and rapid.

165. Based on this information, you would suspect the patient is most likely suffering from which of the following?

   A. intra-abdominal bleeding

   B. pelvic fracture

   C. pneumothorax

   D. bilateral femur fractures

166. The abdominal pain and tenderness in the patient is most likely due to:

   A. blood collecting around the femur.

   B. blood irritating the peritoneal lining.

   C. fecal material causing diaphragmatic irritation.

   D. pleural lining collapse.

167. While you are collecting the SAMPLE history during the focused history and physical exam on a medical patient complaining of dyspnea, the patient states that he feels his breathing is much better when he sits straight up. This is reported as an item addressing what component of the mnemonic OPQRST?

   A. severity

   B. provocation/palliation (alleviation)

   C. radiation

   D. quality

168. Pain on palpation of the symphysis pubis most likely indicates:

   A. a bladder infection.

   B. a ruptured ovary.

   C. a pelvic fracture.

   D. intra-abdominal bleeding.

169. You are transporting a 46-year-old male patient from the scene of an auto crash. He is complaining of pelvic pain and abdominal discomfort. An ongoing assessment should be conducted every:

   A. 30 minutes.

   B. 15 minutes.

   C. 5 minutes.

   D. 2 minutes.

170. A patient with right-side heart failure likely has:

   A. a distended abdomen.

   B. jugular vein distention.

   C. tracheal deviation.

   D. pain to the lower extremities.

171. You are conducting a focused physical exam on a patient complaining of chest pain. Which of the following assessments is *not* included in your examination?

   A. oral mucosa

   B. breath sounds

   C. ears and nose

   D. pedal pulses

172. You have just transported a patient suspected of having suffered a heart attack to the emergency department. Upon your arrival, you are greeted at the door by the emergency department ward clerk who instructs you to place the patient in room B. As you transfer the patient to the hospital bed, you receive a tone from your dispatcher for another emergency call. You should:

   A. immediately leave the emergency department and respond to the call.

   B. wait to notify the nurse or physician of the patient's condition prior to leaving.

   C. refuse to take the call until you have completed your prehospital report.

   D. instruct the ward clerk to pass the information about the patient to the physician.

173. Which of the following is considered a significant mechanism of injury?

   A. a 20-mile-per-hour auto crash

   B. a gunshot wound to the lower leg

   C. a deformed steering wheel in a rear-end collision

   D. a fall of less than twice the patient's height

Scenario

Questions 174–175 refer to the following scenario:

You arrive on the scene and find a patient who fell off a balcony at a hard rock concert. He struck several people when he fell before being impaled on a broken piece of plastic. Upon your arrival at the scene, you note three people lying on the ground next to the patient.

174. As you enter the scene, what is your immediate action?

    A. Perform an primary assessment on each patient to determine who is the most severely injured.

    B. Ask that the police remove all of the people at the concert before approaching the patient.

    C. Call for at least two additional ambulances to respond to the scene.

    D. Go right to the patient impaled on the plastic and begin your assessment.

175. You are now treating the patient impaled on the plastic. You take in-line spinal stabilization and note a large pool of blood around the left thigh where the clothing is soaked in blood. The patient is moaning and groaning in pain. You should immediately:

    A. apply a tourniquet to the leg to stop the bleeding.

    B. expose the extremity to assess for major bleeding.

    C. check the radial pulse to determine whether the patient is in shock.

    D. assess the airway and breathing and apply a nonrebreather mask at 15 lpm.

176. Which of the following indicates a patient priority status?

    A. a 78-year-old patient who cannot remember his name today

    B. warm, dry skin in an patient who is elderly

    C. dizziness and weakness in a patient who is diabetic

    D. a patient with emphysema who presents with a cough

177. A 30-year-old female patient fell off of her bicycle. She was not wearing a helmet. During your detailed physical exam, you notice leakage of clear fluid from her nose. This is most likely a sign of a(n):

    A. infraorbital fracture.

    B. basilar skull fracture.

    C. fractured nose.

    D. zygomatic arch injury.

178. You are treating a two-year-old girl who has been vomiting and suffering diarrhea for the past three days. The best method to assess whether she has lost a significant amount of volume is to:

    A. take a systolic and diastolic blood pressure.

    B. assess the radial pulses and skin color, temperature, and condition.

    C. determine the mental status and whether she is oriented × 3.

    D. inspect the sclera for redness.

179. When conducting the primary assessment, you should always assume that the patient with an altered mental status:

    A. has a head injury.

    B. cannot maintain his own airway.

    C. needs bag-valve-mask ventilation with supplemental oxygen.

    D. will not have radial pulses.

180. You arrive at the scene of a bar fight and find a 25-year-old man who has been stabbed several times and is bleeding severely from a wound to the neck, which is spurting bright red blood. The assailant is still at the bar in the bathroom. You can hear

the sirens of the police who are not yet on the scene. How would you proceed?

A. Try to keep the assailant calm and in the bathroom while you quickly apply direct pressure to the knife wound in the patient's neck.

B. Both you and your partner call out to the assailant to put the knife down so that you can enter the bar to take care of the patient.

C. Remain in the ambulance until the police arrive on the scene and indicate that it is safe to enter.

D. As soon as you see the police cars, quickly enter the scene and apply direct pressure to the wound, and drag the patient to safety.

181. A paradoxical motion of the chest occurs when:

A. a segment moves inward on exhalation.

B. a segment moves outward on exhalation.

C. a segment moves outward on inhalation.

D. a segment does not move with respiration.

182. Stridor is an indication of:

A. a fluid or vomitus obstructing the upper airway.

B. bronchoconstriction and mucus obstructing the lower airway.

C. the tongue blocking the upper airway.

D. laryngeal edema partially occluding the upper airway.

183. You arrive at the scene of a fall and find a 42-year-old woman sitting on the ground next to a ladder. She says she fell only a couple of feet and twisted her ankle. She is complaining of a sharp stabbing pain in her ankle. Which component of the primary assessment must be assessed next in this patient?

A. mental status

B. airway

C. breathing

D. circulation

184. A 62-year-old female patient who has been working in her garden has hot, dry skin. This patient could be suffering from:

A. a heart attack.

B. heat exposure.

C. shock.

D. a stroke.

185. The decision to perform a rapid medical assessment or SAMPLE history first in the medical patient is determined by:

A. the mechanism of injury.

B. the nature of the illness.

C. the signs of medical illness.

D. the patient's mental status.

186. You are assessing a 23-year-old female patient who is complaining of abdominal pain. While you are gathering your history, it is important to ask her which of the following questions?

A. When was the last time you had intercourse?

B. Have you ever smoked crack cocaine?

C. Are you a drug user?

D. When was your last menstrual period?

187. You are assessing a patient complaining of chest pain. You obtain a set of vital signs and find the following: blood pressure, 112/64; heart rate, 112 per minute; and respiration rate, 16 per minute with adequate tidal volume. The pulse oximetry (SpO_2) is 97 percent. You should report that the patient has:

    A. a narrow pulse pressure.
    B. tachypnea.
    C. tachycardia.
    D. hypertension.

188. While assessing the trauma patient, you logroll him and find an open wound to the posterior thorax. You should immediately:

    A. increase the flow of oxygen to 15 lpm.
    B. begin bag-valve-mask ventilation.
    C. assess the lower extremities for other wounds.
    D. apply an occlusive dressing.

189. The medical term for *swelling* is:

    A. erythema.
    B. edema.
    C. ecchymosis.
    D. contusion.

190. Once you have inspected and palpated the neck in the rapid trauma assessment, the next step is to:

    A. inspect the chest.
    B. apply a cervical spinal immobilization collar.
    C. relieve your partner of holding in-line stabilization if the patient has no pain or obvious injury.
    D. auscultate the chest for decreased breath sounds.

191. You arrive on the scene and find a patient who aspirated a large amount of vomitus.

You would expect to find which of the following in the assessment?

    A. pale, cool, clammy skin
    B. cyanosis
    C. constricted pupils
    D. absent breath sounds

192. You arrive on the scene and find a patient who has fallen down the steps. As you approach the patient she states, "I am fine but embarrassed. Just leave me alone and I'll be fine." You should immediately:

    A. take in-line spinal immobilization.
    B. open the airway and check inside the mouth.
    C. have her sign a refusal form.
    D. ask if it is okay to assess her to determine whether she is injured.

193. A patient suffering an allergic reaction most likely has:

    A. crackles.
    B. decreased breath sounds on one side.
    C. wheezing.
    D. gurgling sounds in the upper airway.

194. You arrive on the scene and find a patient who claims that his abdominal pain was less intense following ingestion of an antacid. In your history, you report this as:

    A. provocation or aggravation.
    B. premedication.
    C. palliation or alleviation.
    D. past medical history.

195. Which of the following can be a sign in an unresponsive patient that he could have suffered a seizure?

    A. a rapid radial pulse
    B. an increased systolic blood pressure
    C. poor capillary refill in the nail beds
    D. a lacerated tongue

196. Subcutaneous emphysema most likely indicates which of the following conditions?
    A. myocardial infarction
    B. pericardial tamponade
    C. ruptured aorta
    D. lacerated bronchiole

197. Which of the following assessment components can be skipped because of the patient's condition or estimated time of arrival to the hospital?
    A. primary assessment
    B. focused assessment
    C. ongoing assessment
    D. detailed physical exam

198. A patient with a tension pneumothorax also has:
    A. a widened pulse pressure with a low diastolic blood pressure.
    B. a decreased heart rate and weak peripheral pulses.
    C. warm, dry skin that is moist to touch.
    D. a decreased systolic blood pressure.

199. An primary assessment must be conducted on:
    A. only patients who present with an altered mental status.
    B. all patients with either an illness or injury.
    C. those patients who would require an immediate intervention.
    D. patients when time and patient condition permits.

200. A 26-year-old female patient is found responsive and alert at the scene of a car rollover. She complains of upper abdominal pain. Following an appropriate patient assessment, you decide to transport. En route she becomes less responsive. Her breathing rate increases. As a part of your ongoing assessment, you should immediately:
    A. repeat a focused history and physical exam.
    B. repeat a detailed physical exam.
    C. repeat the primary assessment.
    D. contact medical direction.

201. The purpose of the rapid trauma assessment is to:
    A. identify and manage life threats to the patient.
    B. locate all injuries to the patient.
    C. assess the airway, breathing, and circulatory status.
    D. identify injuries that will require surgical interventions.

202. Which of the following signs indicates that the patient is having trouble breathing?
    A. The patient talks in a normal speech pattern.
    B. The patient is crying vigorously.
    C. The patient says a few words and gasps for a breath.
    D. The patient complains that his throat feels as though it is closing.

203. You are treating a 28-year-old female who fell 20 feet while roofing a house. After determining that she is unresponsive, you would immediately:
    A. open her airway using a head-tilt, chin-lift maneuver.
    B. apply in-line stabilization and open her airway.
    C. start high concentration oxygen using a nonrebreather mask.
    D. open her airway and start high concentration oxygen.

204. You are treating a 78-year-old female patient who was found at home on the living room floor by her daughter. She is unresponsive to painful stimuli. Her respirations are 15 per minute with very minimal chest wall movement. What should you do first?

A. Apply a nonrebreather mask at 15 lpm and assess the pulse.

B. Provide two ventilations and reassess the mental status.

C. Immediately move the patient to the ambulance and begin transport.

D. Insert an oropharyngeal airway and begin bag-valve-mask ventilation.

205. During palpation of the abdomen in the rapid trauma assessment, the patient makes a facial grimace and draws his knees upward. You would note this as abdominal:

A. rigidity.

B. tenderness.

C. guarding.

D. pain.

✓answers
& rationales

1.

C. The scene survey should begin as you are pulling up to the scene. You should identify potential hazards (fire, downed power lines, gas leaks) and look for clues to identify an unsafe scene (all the lights off in the house, general atmosphere of the scene, listening for arguing or fighting) before leaving the ambulance.

2.

D. All of the scenes listed potentially present a hazard or could rapidly deteriorate to a hazardous scene. However, scenes that involve patients who change their behavior very rapidly are most likely to turn violent and injure the EMT. These scenes usually involve patients who are intoxicated, under the influence of drugs, or have behavioral disorders. Typically in crime scenes involving shootings and stabbings, the perpetrator is gone prior to EMS arrival.

3.

B. All power lines are considered energized until a power company representative arrives on the scene and advises you they are not. Downed power lines pose a serious threat to rescuers and the public. You should advise the patients to remain inside the vehicle until you can safely remove them. Never try to move power lines. Those that are on the ground can energize the area around them. Keep a safe distance away.

4.

C. If at any time you feel the scene is not safe, you and your partner should attempt to make it safe or retreat until the proper resources make the scene safe. There is no reason to assess this scene further. You have already determined that it is unsafe. Do not make contact with bystanders or the patient until the police secure the scene.

5.

A. In a closed environment like a house when more than one patient complains of the same symptoms, you should suspect a toxic environment such as carbon monoxide poisoning. Clues that lead you to suspect a toxic environment in this situation include winter morning (furnace use), inside the house (enclosed space), and more than one patient with the same symptoms.

6.

D. Of the scenes listed, a bar is the most likely place for the EMT to be injured. Calls to bars may or may not involve a police response. These calls often involve intoxicated patients who have a tendency to change their behavior rapidly.

7.

A. Your first and foremost responsibility at the crime scene is to provide emergency medical care. If possible, prevent the destruction of evidence by not touching weapons and preventing unnecessary personnel from entering the crime scene. Your own personal safety is the ultimate priority.

8.

C. Upon arriving at a crash scene, assess and observe the entire scene. Do not focus on the vehicles or patients involved. Look to the right of, left of, above, and below the vehicle to ensure a safe scene. Remember that the area encompassing an accident scene can extend hundreds of feet in high-speed crashes.

9.

B. You cannot determine whether a patient is oriented by simple eye openings in response to verbal stimuli. The patient is reported to respond to verbal stimuli.

10.

B. During the scene size-up upon your arrival, you attempt to categorize the call as medical or trauma. As you continue the scene size-up and primary assessment, you continue determining whether the patient is experiencing a traumatic injury or a medical illness. In some scenes, you may not be able to determine the patient's true etiology and will not be able to categorize the patient. Also, some calls categorize the patient as both a trauma and a medical patient. As an example, if you arrive on the scene for an elderly patient who has an obviously fractured hip, you need to determine the reason for the fracture. If the patient states that he tripped over the carpet and fell, he would be categorized as a trauma patient. If the patient states that he does not remember or that he got dizzy and then fell, the patient would be categorized as both trauma (due to the fall) and medical (due to the dizziness). If you arrive on the scene and the patient is not responding, you will not be able to determine whether the injury was solely due to a fall or other traumatic event and therefore categorize the patient as both trauma and medical.

11.

B. Falls, motor vehicle crashes, and shootings all involve injury or the potential for physical injury due to the mechanism of injury. Sometimes it is obvious, and at other times, you must search for it. If you encounter a patient who is unresponsive and the call has an unknown circumstance, consider both a traumatic injury and medical illness in the patient. You would attempt to identify a potential mechanism of injury to as a cause for the unresponsiveness.

12.

A. When you arrive at a scene and determine that there are more patients than you can effectively manage, immediately call for additional assistance. This is often done before exiting the ambulance, immediately after entering the scene, and before making patient contact. If you make patient contact before calling for additional assistance, you could become focused on that one patient rather than the whole scene. It is most important to get the necessary resources to the scene as early as possible, thus, the decision is typically made during the scene size-up.

13.

D. Determining the total number of patients is a major element of the scene size-up. Try to do this before making patient contact. The total number of patients determines how many additional resources are needed.

14.
D. Regardless how severely injured the patients are, it is necessary to get additional assistance to the scene as quickly as possible. Requesting additional resources is typically done as part of the scene size-up and before any patient contact. Immediately loading one patient and beginning transport is not appropriate and could put you at risk of abandoning the other patients.

15.
C. The general overall impression is based on the findings at the scene and the mechanism of injury. These two assessments allow you to categorize your patient into medical or trauma categories and determine the priority of care.

16.
A. Nonpurposeful movement has relationship to the painful (tactile) stimulation. A purposeful movement is one in which the patient makes an active attempt to remove the source of painful stimulation. There are two types of nonpurposeful movement. *Decorticate (flexion) posturing* occurs when the patient arches the back and flexes his arms toward the chest. *Decerebrate (extension) posturing* occurs when the patient arches the back and extends his arms parallel to the body.

17.
B. An alert adult who is gasping for air, is unable to speak, coughs excessively, or has stridor indicates a partial airway obstruction. Talking in complete sentences and crying or drooling can indicate simply a sore throat.

18.
B. If you suspect the patient could have an injured spine, you must provide in-line spinal stabilization prior to continuing with the assessment. The patient could have fallen down the stairs. If you were to ask the patient questions before stabilizing the spine, he will likely look toward you, thus compromising the spine.

19.
D. The most effective way to determine whether the depth of breathing is adequate is by looking at the patient's chest for chest rise and fall and listening and feeling for air exchange over his mouth and nose.

20.
A. Your initial action for an apneic patient is to provide immediate positive pressure ventilation. Delaying positive pressure ventilation likely results in brain damage or cardiac arrest. This patient was found lying in bed and spinal injury is not suspected.

21.
B. After ensuring an adequate airway, assess the patient's breathing status. If you are in doubt as to the breathing adequacy, provide positive pressure ventilation. Applying a gauze pad is not appropriate for an open chest wound.

22.
C. The patient could be presenting with a sign of a tension pneumothorax, a serious chest injury. Immediately auscultate for absent breath sounds and check for additional signs such as jugular venous distention (JVD) and a tracheal deviation. You also should release the occlusive dressing that is covering the sucking chest wound. If breath sounds, JVD, and/or tracheal shift are not present, you should recheck the airway and ensure proper head position.

23.
D. The patient is potentially suffering from a head injury and requires hyperventilation at 20 ventilations per minute if he is displaying signs of brain herniation such as a fixed and dilated pupil, nonpurposeful posturing, and paralysis to one side. Cover the right ear loosely with a sterile dressing.

24.
D. Your initial response to an obstructed airway from a foreign body in the infant is to deliver five rapid back blows while supporting his body over your hand and knee. Chest thrusts are delivered after the back blows. Never administer abdominal thrusts to an infant. Blind finger sweeps are not performed on the infant because this procedure could lodge the foreign body farther into the airway.

25.
B. Current research has found that the location of perfusing pulses does not accurately estimate systolic blood pressures.

26.
B. In the adult patient, you first palpate the radial pulse, whereas in an infant, assess the brachial artery in the upper arm. The carotid artery in the adult and femoral artery in the infant are assessed when the peripheral pulses are absent.

27.
A. Blood flowing from a wound at a steady continuous flow is considered major bleeding. You should immediately apply direct pressure to the wound with a gloved hand. Most bleeding can be controlled by direct pressure. Once the bleeding has been controlled, you should apply a pressure dressing.

28.
D. Hot, cool, and cold skin temperatures are considered abnormal. Hot skin usually indicates hyperthermia (heat emergency) or an infection. Cold skin is found in hypothermia (cold emergency), and cool skin is usually a sign of hypoperfusion (shock).

29.
C. Capillary refill can be assessed in all patients; however, it is most reliable in younger patients who do not have a pre-existing disease. Capillary refill is most reliable in the infant or child less than six years of age. It can be quickly checked in the nail bed, the fleshy part of the palm along the ulnar margin, forehead, or cheeks. Capillary refill is usually less than 2 seconds, it is influenced by cold temperature in patients of all ages. Thus, if the patient is in a cold environment, the vasoconstriction of the vessels in the skin would cause the capillary refill to be delayed regardless of the volume of blood.

30.
A. The mechanism of injury could not be very apparent or well understood upon arrival at the scene. You should reconsider the mechanism of injury during the secondary to re-evaluate whether it was enough to be considered significant.

31.
B. Falls, if of more than 10 feet, bicycle collisions, and vehicle collisions in which a person in the same passenger compartment of the patient has died are all considered significant. Low-speed motor vehicle collisions are not considered significant.

32.
A. The patient with a significant mechanism of injury requires a rapid trauma assessment to include baseline vitals and then a SAMPLE history.

33.
A. The first step in the assessment of any patient following scene size-up is to perform an primary assessment. This is followed by the rapid trauma assessment if a significant mechanism of injury is suspected. Taking baseline vital signs and a SAMPLE history are included in the secondary assessment..

34.
B. The rapid trauma assessment is a quick head-to-toe exam performed on patients with a significant mechanism of injury or altered mental status. It is conducted to identify critical injuries.

The focused trauma assessment is performed when you do not have a significant mechanism of injury or altered mental status and is focused on a specific injury. The SAMPLE history is performed at the end of the rapid trauma assessment. Assessment of the baseline vital signs is obtained at the end of the rapid trauma assessment.

35.
C. The type of assessment that is performed on a trauma patient is based on the mechanism of injury and primary assessment findings.

36.
D. Immediately perform a rapid trauma assessment to determine whether a life-threatening injury or condition exists.

37.
D. A rapid head-to-toe assessment that is performed on the injured or ill patient to identify life-threatening injuries is *a rapid trauma assessment.*

38.
C. A patient who has a significant mechanism of injury, an altered mental status, or the possibility of having multiple injuries requires a rapid trauma assessment. Because this patient is not oriented to place, he is considered to have an altered mental status and needs rapid trauma assessment to identify any potential life threats.

39.
C. DCAP-BTLS is the mnemonic for deformities, contusions, abrasions, punctures, burns, tenderness, lacerations, and swelling. These are signs of injury that should be identified during your rapid trauma assessment.

40.
C. The rapid trauma assessment is conducted to identify potential life-threatening injuries to the patient. It uses a systematic approach, starting at the head and proceeding down the neck, chest, abdomen, pelvis, lower extremities, upper extremities, and finally the posterior body.

41.
C. Palpate the entire head and face, noting any tenderness or deformities. The immobilization device should not be removed to perform a detailed physical exam. Gently palpate the skull with your hands flattened over the skull to prevent inadvertently pushing your finger tips into a skull fracture.

42.
D. If you find inadequate breathing while performing a rapid trauma assessment, you must immediately stop the assessment and provide positive pressure ventilation. Management of the airway and breathing takes precedence over continued assessment.

43.
A. Paradoxical chest wall movement associated with a flail segment indicates a critical injury affecting the patient's breathing and must be managed immediately. It is normal to find flat jugular veins with a patient sitting at a 45° angle. Flat jugular veins in the supine patient could indicate a decreased blood volume. An open humerus fracture, unless it is associated with major bleeding, is not considered a life-threatening injury, nor is a tibia fracture.

44.
B. The rapid trauma assessment is performed to determine whether additional life-threatening injuries or conditions are present. Subsequent care and treatment are based on this examination.

45.
A. No mechanism of injury in a medical patient will tell you about your patient's injuries. Therefore, you must become a detective and look for any and all clues about the chief complaint.

Further assessment of the chief complaint is considered the history of the present illness.

46.
D. The OPQRST mnemonic helps you to rapidly and systematically gather more information about the chief complaint.

47.
B. The mnemonic OPQRST stands for onset, provocation, quality, radiation, severity, and time length that the patient has had the symptom.

48.
A. *Provocation* determines what makes the symptom worse, whereas *palliation* determines what makes the symptom better. This provides the EMT the information to help gauge the severity of the patient's illness.

49.
B. This question refers to radiation of pain. The question is assessing whether the pain or symptom moves or radiates.

50.
A. When assessing the quality of a patient's pain, you should ask open-ended questions, such as "What does the pain feel like?" Asking leading questions, such as "Is the pain sharp or dull?" can lead to an inaccurate description. Questions regarding what makes the pain worse pertain to provocation, not quality. Asking questions about when and how the pain began pertains to onset.

51.
A. Gather the history first in the responsive medical patient. The history provides valuable information and must be obtained before the patient becomes potentially unresponsive. The history is followed by the making a focused exam and taking vital signs.

52.
C. In the unresponsive medical patient, perform a rapid medical assessment to determine the nature of the medical illness. This is followed by taking the vital signs and patient history.

53.
C. The unresponsive medical patient is considered a high-priority patient. Unresponsiveness is a critical finding.

54.
B. Valuable information is commonly obtained when inspecting the area around the unresponsive medical patient. The condition of the patient's environment, presence of home oxygen supply, the patient's position in a hospital bed, and patient's medications are a few examples of things that could provide information about the patient or his past medical history.

55.
B. Unequal pupils usually indicate stroke or possible head injury. Changes in pupil size and reactivity are commonly associated with drug overdose, oxygen starvation (hypoxia), or adverse environmental conditions.

56.
D. When you have determined that your patient is unresponsive or has an altered mental status during the primary assessment, your next assessment step is to perform a rapid medical assessment. It will help to determine the nature of the medical illness. The status of the airway, breathing, and circulation is assessed and managed during the primary assessment.

57.
D. The unresponsive medical patient should be placed in the lateral recumbent position, also known as the *recovery* or *coma position*. This position helps to protect the airway from vomitus, blood, and other secretions. Be prepared to

suction the airway if secretions are present. The Trendelenburg (shock) position helps increase blood perfusion to the brain and vital organs. The semi-Fowler's position requires the patient to sit at a semireclined position, which could permit secretions and vomitus to enter the airway and lungs. The prone position (face down) will not permit access to the patient's face and airway.

58.
B. You will initially assess the responsive medical patient by evaluating the complaint and signs and symptoms by using the mnemonic OPQRST. Perform a rapid medical assessment on patients you find unresponsive. In the responsive medical patient, perform components of a secondary assessment after you make a transport decision. You should perform a focused medical exam in the responsive patient after you obtain a SAMPLE history.

59.
A. The secondary assessment is performed after all life-threatening injuries have been managed. During the secondary assessment the EMT should identify and treat all nonlife-threatening wounds or injuries.

60.
D. At the scene of a trauma, the scene size-up, primary assessment, and rapid trauma assessment are performed. After the patient has been loaded into the ambulance, perform an ongoing assessment. If time and the patient's condition permit, a detailed secondary assessment is then performed to identify all nonlife-threatening injuries.

61.
A. During the detailed secondary assessment, many of the same components of the rapid trauma assessment are reassessed. However, the detailed physical exam is designed to allow the EMT to perform a more thorough exam of certain areas of the body. The eyes would be assessed in more detail and the conjunctiva would be assessed.

62.
B. A yellow color in the white portion of the eye (sclera) is called *icterus* and indicates possible liver damage or failure.

63.
B. Trauma to the trachea, bronchi, bronchioles, lungs, or esophagus can cause subcutaneous emphysema, the term that describes trapped air under the skin. Trapped air under the skin can be palpated and feels like crackling or crepitation. Monitor the patient closely for evidence of respiratory distress.

64.
A. *Paradoxical movement* is the term used to describe the chest wall that moves inward during inhalation and outward during exhalation. This type of movement indicates a flail segment. This is a true emergency and must be treated immediately. Often flail segments can be missed during the primary or rapid trauma assessment because the area is stabilized by muscle spasm. The major life-threatening problem associated with a flail segment is the potential for an underlying pulmonary contusion.

65.
B. Any injuries found during the detailed physical exam are managed as discovered. Lacerations are bandaged and fractures immobilized.

66.
D. A trauma patient who is unable to close his mouth most likely has suffered a fracture or dislocation of the mandible. The most important concern is to closely observe the patient's airway to prevent obstruction and possible aspiration.

67.
C. Do not remove any foreign body embedded in the eye or force the eyelids open in the presence of an eyelid injury. Pressure should not be used

to control bleeding from the eyeball. Both pupils should respond and react simultaneously to a light source. This is called a *consensual reflex.*

68.
B. Pupils that are large in size and do not respond to light are termed *fixed* and *dilated.*

69.
C. *Visual acuity* is clarity of vision. *Conjugate movement* describes the eyes moving together as a unit. A *conjugate gaze* is a gaze or stare in which both eyes are looking in the same direction.

70.
D. A patient with a fixed and dilated pupil who is alert and oriented could have sustained a direct injury to the eye. Other possibilities include the presence of a glass eye, a localized nerve injury, or the use of eye drops such as atropine or pilocarpine that dilate the pupils. If the pupil is fixed and dilated as a result of a head injury and brain herniation, the patient would not be alert and oriented. The brain has to be herniated deeply into the skull before the pupil becomes fixed and dilated. This would not allow the patient to remain alert and oriented.

71.
D. Air trapped under the skin can be caused by a tension pneumothorax called *subcutaneous emphysema.* It can crackle and cause a sound called *crepitation.* It can result from a trauma to the respiratory tract, airway, lung, or esophagus.

72.
D. The oral mucosa is very vascular and reflects a patient's perfusion status. Pale oral mucosa typically indicates that the patient has been bleeding over a long period of time such as in a gastrointestinal bleed. The patient with an acute bleed usually does not present with a severely pale oral mucosa.

73.
D. The presence of wheezes during auscultation typically indicates constriction and inflammation of the bronchioles in the lower airway. Wheezing produces a high-pitched sound usually heard on exhalation early and inhalation as the constriction and inflammation progresses. Ronchi, which produce a snoring type of sound indicate the presence of mucous in the larger airways. As the bronchioles constrict and become inflamed, the airway resistance increases. The trachea and bronchi are supported by hard cartilage rings that do not allow them to constrict.

74.
A. One of the purposes of the ongoing assessment is to determine whether the patient's condition is improving or deteriorating. The primary assessment is repeated in addition to checking the interventions performed and to further assessing or repeating the assessment of areas of new complaint. The focused secondary assessment is designed to inspect particular areas of the body. The ongoing assessment is not designed to identify initial life threats, which should have been identified in the rapid trauma assessment. If life-threatening injuries are being missed in the rapid trauma assessment, the EMT is not performing a competent rapid trauma assessment.

75.
B. All critically injured patients should be reassessed at least every five minutes so that indicators of a worsening situation or an improvement can be noted rapidly. Stable patients are reassessed every 15 minutes.

76.
D. Any change in the patient's condition or complaint would cause you to perform an onging assessment. Because the patient has a new complaint, you would assess the abdomen even if it had been assessed previously.

77.

D. The primary assessment evaluates life threats to the airway, breathing, and circulation. The airway is opened by a manual maneuver. When assessing the breathing status of the patient, both the respiratory rate and depth of breathing must be checked to a determine whether the breathing is adequate. If only the respiratory rate or depth of breathing is known, you cannot make a decision whether to ventilate the patient. It takes two adequates—adequate rate and adequate depth—to categorize the breathing status as adequate. It takes only one inadequate—inadequate rate or inadequate depth—to categorize the breathing status as inadequate. Inadequate respiration requires ventilation.

78.

D. The information gathered from a repeated assessment should always be compared with previous findings to identify trends in the patient's condition. This helps to determine the patient's current status, know whether the treatment you are providing is helping the patient, and quickly identify a deteriorating patient status.

79.

C. The patient has not suffered a significant mechanism of injury, altered mental status, or multiple injuries. Thus, you can do a focused physical exam on the injured foot. Perform baseline vital signs as part of the secondary. An ongoing assessment is conducted every 15 minutes in this patient because he is considered to be stable.

80.

B. If there is a change in the pateint's status, conduct an ongoing assessment. One of the first components of it is the reassessment of the mental status using the AVPU mnemonic. Because the patient is no longer alert, the next thing you would do is to determine whether she responds to verbal stimuli. Simply ask her to open her eyes. If she does not respond, move to a trapez-ius pinch to determine whether she responds to painful stimuli. You would then continue with the primary assessment to determine the need to open the airway or ventilate the patient.

81.

B. A decrease in the pulse rate and pulse quality can indicate a head injury or severe hypoxia. These signs should alert you to other injuries or the need to change your treatment, such as providing positive pressure ventilation. A low blood sugar level (hypoglycemia) usually presents with an increased heart rate. A heat-related emergency usually presents with an increased heart rate that can be very strong. As the condition continues, the heart rate remains high and the quality becomes poor. An allergic reaction (anaphylactic shock) presents with an increased heart rate that can be of poor quality.

82.

A. An ongoing assessment is made to detect any changes in the patient's condition, to detect any missed injuries or conditions, and to adjust treatment as needed. If the patient has any abnormal findings in the primary assessment, you should perform an ongoing assessment every 5 minutes.

83.

D. By waiting at least 1 full second before you speak into the microphone, you are allowing time for the repeater to "open" the channel, preventing the initial part of your transmission from being cut off.

84.

B. By saying "Over," you are informing the receiver that you have finished your transmission. By waiting for confirmation, you have assurance that the other party got your message and has no more questions.

85.

C. Using a standard format when communicating to medical direction is very helpful. Use the following sequence: (1) your unit number and level of service, (2) the patient's age and sex, (3) the patient's chief complaint, (4) a brief history of the present illness, including scene assessment and mechanism of injury, (5) major past history, (6) patient's mental status, (7) patient's baseline vital signs, (8) pertinent findings of your physical exam, (9) description of the medical care you have administered, and (10) the patient's response to the emergency medical care.

86.
A. After medical direction has given you an order, you should repeat the order back to medical direction word for word. Repeating the order back, referred to as the echo method, helps ensure that the order was given and received correctly. If the person giving you the order has not identified himself, you should ask for his name and document it on the run report.

87.
D. Be sure that the information you provide is accurate and is reported clearly. A patient's life can depend on the decisions that are made. If you do not understand an order, ask that it be repeated. Repeat back critical information to medical direction.

88.
C. The oral report should summarize only the information you have already given the staff: any changes that have occurred, current vital signs, and any treatment rendered. The oral report should not be a duplicate of your radio report.

89.
B. By establishing yourself at the same or lower level of the patient, you help decrease his fear and anxiety.

90.
C. Do not offend older patients by automatically assuming that you have to raise your voice when speaking to them or by rushing the patients' thoughts or actions. Many patients need more

time to reflect on the question and form a response. Allow him enough time to adequately respond to the question.

91.
B. Effective communication of patient information is important in the oral report because it allows hospital personnel to provide for a smooth transition of care. Provide the hospital personnel with your unit's ID number, patient's age/sex, chief complaint, brief pertinent history, major past illness, mental status, vital signs, physical exam findings, care provided and response to this care, and your estimated arrival time at the facility.

92.
C. Push the press to talk button and wait 1 second before transmitting. Speak with your mouth 2 to 3 inches from the microphone. After receiving orders from medical direction, echo back the orders. Avoid making a diagnosis and provide only objective information or im-portant relevant subjective information.

93.
B. The Federal Communications Commission is responsible for licensing base station operations, assigning call signs, approving equipment for use, limiting transmitter power output, and monitoring field operations.

94.
C. Cellular telephone use in EMS is common. The major disadvantage is that these telephones are part of the public telephone system that can easily be overwhelmed in a multiple casualty disaster.

95.
C. A repeater takes a low-power signal, changes the frequency, and increases the power of the signal. Repeaters are common in large areas or where the terrain makes transmission and reception of signals difficult.

96.

A. CAD refers to *computer aided dispatch.*

97.

A. The EMT must accurately transcribe and record response times when obtained from the emergency medical dispatcher. These times can become vitally important if the call should lead to a court case. The EMT must take the times from the dispatch and accurately transcribe them on the patient care report.

98.

D. The Federal Communications Commission (FCC) has jurisdiction over all radio operations in the United States. This includes EMS and other public service radios.

99.

B. Anytime you believe an order is inappropriate, it is best to question the order. Medical direction could have misunderstood the patient information that you provided. Questioning the order can prevent the administration of a harmful medication or performance of an inappropriate procedure.

100.

D. If medical direction has given you an order that you believe is outside your scope of practice, you should immediately question it. It is possible that medical direction misunderstood something you said or misspoke when giving the order. If medical direction continues to insist that you perform the order, disregard the order and continue to treat the patient within your scope of practice. Be sure to inform your supervisor and document the event.

101.

C. Often patients are under a tremendous amount of stress. Speaking calmly and slowly helps to engender the patient's confidence in you and reduce his stress. You should raise your voice only if the patient is hard of hearing. Avoid medical terms. Speak so the patient can understand you. Do not use codes because doing so can elevate the patient's stress. Be truthful to the patient and speak so he can understand what is happening.

102.

D. The Department of Transportation determined that this was the minimum to be written on all run reports. Remember that accurate documentation helps prevent any questions or problems later.

103.

C. The Department of Transportation requires times that relate only to the specific call (time to dispatch, response time, time to patient side, on-scene time, and transport time). After arriving on the scene, the next communication occurs when you arrive at the patient's side.

104.

B. The following is the minimum data set that the Department of Transportation requires: chief complaint, level of responsiveness, systolic blood pressure, skin perfusion, skin color and temperature, pulse rate, and respiratory rate and effort.

105.

A. The patient narrative section of the patient care report includes the chief complaint, SAMPLE history, and/or the description of the mechanism of injury. The patient's name, age, sex, and blood pressure are parts of the patient data section, not the narrative section.

106.

A. *QID* is the acceptable abbreviation for four times a day. For example, the patient is prescribed a bronchodilator treatment QID. *SOB* is the only acceptable abbreviation for shortness of breath. *TID* is the abbreviation for three times a day. *NTG* is the abbreviation for nitroglycerin.

107.

C. The Department of Transportation established the minimum data set to standardize information collected by EMS systems. It allows for comparisons between and among systems and improvements in care.

108.

A. Clocks should be synchronized to the dispatch clocks so that time-critical events can be accurately documented. Ideally, at least two sets of vital signs should be obtained. This provides a basis for determining the trend of the vital signs. A diagnosis is not made or reported. Patient information can be shared only with health care providers directly involved in the patient's care.

109.

A. A *pertinent negative* is a complaint that the patient should exhibit but denies having. For example, the patient complains of substernal chest pains but denies the presence of shortness of breath. The patient with AMI type chest pain frequently exhibits shortness of breath. It is pertinent to document this absence of symptom.

110.

D. Falsification of the patient care report is *never* acceptable. It can lead to poor continuity of patient care. Knowingly providing false information can lead to the revocation of an EMT certification or license.

111.

C. Documentation of patient refusals requires careful and complete documentation of your efforts to provide care and transport for the patient. Issues related to the determination of the patient's competency at the time are frequently the areas that are contested. Fully document the patient's competency or lack of competency in the patient care report.

112.

D. Confidentiality of patient care report information is important, and you, as the primary EMS field provider, must maintain it. This information cannot be shared with others who are not directly involved in the patient's care. Generally, the only individuals who are allowed access to this information are police officers for an investigation, health care workers for continuity of care, those with a legal subpoena, and third-party billing information. The information officer controls the confidentiality of the information once the patient care report has been submitted to the EMS agency.

113.

D. The EMT needs to have proof that the victim actually refuse transport. Without a signature, it is the victim's word against that of you and your partner.

114.

D. If the EMT suspects that the patient is suffering from any disease or injury or has taken any drug or other substance that can alter the patient's judgment, the EMT can be held liable if he does not treat the patient or arrange for the patient's treatment. The EMT must be sure that the patient is competent and able to make a rational decision. If you are unsure, contact medical direction for assistance.

115.

C. This EMT should offer suggestions on how to gain care or call EMS back to the scene if the patient wants to go to the hospital. When the EMT offers this help, the patient should not feel stranded and helpless.

116.

B. When you make an error on the patient care report, you should draw a single horizontal line through the mistake. The correct information should be written next to the error. Finally, you should initial the information that was corrected.

Any other means of correcting an error could be perceived as a deception or an attempt to cover up a mistake. Remember that the report you write today will be your memory years later when you are called into court.

117.

D. While gathering your general impression of the injured patient, you must manage any life threats before proceeding with the assessment. An open wound to the chest must be immediately managed by placing your gloved hand directly over the wound site.

118.

D. Gunshot entrance wounds can be away from the spine; however, after the projectile enters the body, it can strike the spine. While forming your general impression of this patient before continuing your assessment, you must provide in-line stabilization of the spine.

119.

B. When the mechanism of injury is significant, as it is with this patient, you should perform a rapid secondary assessment of the patient. It is a complete head-to-toe exam that is performed quickly. It helps to identify other injuries such as additional gunshot wounds or exit wounds. The focused physical exam, the exam of the specific injury site, is completed when you do not suspect a significant mechanism of injury.

120.

C. Although doing so seems quite innocent when you are providing care for a patient with a minor injury, you should *never* falsify a patient record. Document the incident accordingly.

121.

A. This is an example of subjective information, which is based on the patient's perceptions or expressions of information that you cannot see or feel. Subjective information is described in the patient care report in the patient narrative section.

122.

D. This is a rather minor example of maintaining patient confidentiality. Confidentiality is the patient's legal right, and it is your ethical responsibility not to divulge such information.

123.

B. The next immediate step in the assessment process is to determine whether the patient responds to verbal stimuli. At this point, you have determined only that he is not alert. He could respond to your voice or command with appropriate communication that would provide information about his airway and breathing status. If he talks to you, there is no need to open the airway manually or to insert an airway adjunct. If he does not respond to verbal stimuli, you then assess his response to painful stimuli. The pulse and skin check occurs after assessment of the breathing status.

124.

B. During the general impression of the primary assessment, you inspect for obvious life-threatening injuries that need immediate management. Upon your approach to the patient, if you note a major bleed, such as spurting or steady flowing blood, you or a partner should quickly expose the area and apply direct pressure. Once direct pressure has been applied, you should then perform the remainder of the primary assessment. Positive pressure ventilation is necessary in this patient; however, it should be performed after establishing the airway. Manual spinal stabilization is necessary and should be performed prior to establishing an airway. Oxygen administration is necessary; however, it will be delivered by positive pressure ventilation. A nonrebreather mask is not appropriate in this patient because it will not provide ventilation.

125.
A. Several life threats must be managed in this patient: the open wound to the chest, the blood in the mouth, the hypoxia, and the poor ventilation status. You must clear the airway immediately— prior to providing positive pressure ventilation—to prevent aspiration. Do not apply a nonrebreather mask until after assessing the ventilation status. In this patient, it appears that the ventilatory status is poor; therefore, oxygen should be delivered via the ventilation device. The gunshot wound to the chest must be occluded as quickly as possible.

126.
A. All of the possible choices are signs or symptoms of a possible fracture. However, the most objective is crepitation, which is a grating sensation found when bone ends rub over each other. Pain, ecchymosis (discoloration), and edema (swelling) could all be found in ligament, tendon, or muscle injuries when there is no actual bone injury.

127.
A. Capillary refill does not provide accurate information in the adult patient as it does in the infant and young child. The adult patient could have pre-existing disease conditions that can cause a delay. Research has found that some people have a normally slow capillary refill, some up to 4 seconds. Also, environmental conditions play a role in capillary refill. A cold environment, for example, causes the refill to be delayed.

128.
C. During the general impression when you are attempting to ascertain the chief complaint, note the patient's speech pattern. A patient who says a few words and then gasps for a breath is showing objective signs of respiratory distress. It is normal for a patient who is crying loudly to gasp for a breath. Typically, patients who are dyspneic sit upright or can be propped up in bed with a few pillows. The fact that the patient is on 2 lpm of oxygen at home does not necessarily mean that he is dyspneic.

129.
B. Because the respirations are shallow, indicating an inadequate tidal volume of air being breathed in, the priority of this patient's management is to establish an airway by employing a jaw-thrust maneuver followed by positive pressure ventilation. Application of a nonrebreather mask will not correct the inadequate tidal volume and will lead to severe hypoxia. Do not take a blood pressure until after the airway and ventilation have been managed and the primary assessment and rapid trauma assessment have been completed. It is more important to establish an airway prior to ventilation than to apply a dressing to a moderately bleeding wound. Only severe bleeding is managed during the primary assessment.

130.
D. Because the patient has the potential for multiple injuries based on the mechanism of injury, a rapid trauma assessment must be conducted. A focused physical exam is used only if there is no possible chance of other injuries. A detailed exam can be conducted after the rapid trauma assessment. The patient should not be transported until after you perform the appropriate assessment and immobilizing the patient to a backboard.

131.
B. All of the choices must be performed on this patient; however, the first priority is to ensure your own safety. Do not get drawn into dramatic scenes without first conducting a scene size-up to be sure safety hazards have been identified and managed.

132.
C. The airway has been secured; therefore, the next immediate action is to begin positive pressure ventilation. Even though the rate is adequate, the tidal volume is not. An inadequate rate or tidal volume indicates inadequate breathing, which is treated by providing positive pressure ventilation. Application of a nonrebreather mask

will provide an increased amount of oxygen to the patient; however, most of the oxygen will not reach the alveoli because the volume is inadequate. Chest compressions are not indicated because the patient still has pulses. A cervical spinal immobilization collar is applied during the rapid trauma assessment, not during the primary assessment.

133.
A. The patient is complaining orally when you arrive on the scene; therefore, you can assume that her airway is open and breathing is adequate. These are both parts of the primary assessment. To complete the primary assessment, assess the circulation by checking the pulses and skin. Because the patient is responsive, you should next obtain a SAMPLE history as part of the secondary for the medical patient.

134.
B. Because the patient is a minor, consent becomes an issue of concern. However, because the patient has suffered a critical injury, it is necessary to initiate emergency care and transport under implied consent. In the case of a minor injury, attempting to contact the parents or legal guardian of the child prior to transport would be prudent.

135.
A. During the general impression of the primary assessment, it is necessary to manage any obvious major bleeding. Because the patient has identified the bleeding, you should quickly assess the foot and determine whether the bleeding is spurting or flowing steadily from the wound. If it is, you must then control the bleeding. If not, you should proceed with the primary assessment and assess the circulation because the airway is patent and breathing is adequate evidenced by the patient's oral complaints and speech pattern.

136.
D. Following the primary assessment, you should next perform a rapid medical assessment

because the patient has an altered mental status. If the patient were coherent, it is appropriate to conduct a focused history and physical exam.

137.
C. You would approach the patient from the front of the vehicle if possible and instruct the patient not to move his head or neck. You or your partner would then gain access to the vehicle and provide manual stabilization of the spine while in the vehicle. Once that has been done, you should then proceed with the general impression and the remainder of the primary assessment.

138.
B. Tracheal deviation and jugular venous distension are late signs of a tension pneumothorax, which occurs from an injury to the pleural lining. Tension pneumothorax allows a large amount of air to enter the pleural space, resulting in a buildup of pressure in the injured side of the chest and causing compression of the mediastinum. This compresses the heart and great vessels, resulting in a decrease in blood pressure, an increase in heart rate, and a narrow pulse pressure. The patient will complain of severe shortness of breath and display signs of respiratory distress. The perfusion and respiratory signs, along with severely decreased or absent breath sounds on the injured side, are much earlier signs of a tension pneumothorax.

139.
C. The patient obviously has an altered mental status; therefore, he could be deemed unable to make a rational decision. Based on implied consent, you should assess the patient, begin emergency care, and transport the patient.

140.
D. Capillary refill is most accurate in younger children. It is used to assess the patient's perfusion status. Capillary refill is subject to environmental influences such as cold weather that would cause the vessels in the periphery to

constrict, thereby reducing the blood flow to that area, causing the capillary refill to be reduced. The asthma patient is suffering a ventilation problem, not a perfusion problem. It is appropriate to assess capillary refill in the 30-year-old who was shot in the chest; however, it has been found that the capillary refill test is most accurate in younger children.

141.

A. Blood mixed with clear fluid coming from the ears, nose, or mouth is likely blood mixed with cerebrospinal fluid. This is typically an indication of a skull fracture. A "halo test" can be performed to determine whether the blood is mixed with cerebrospinal fluid by dropping blood onto a cotton gauze pad or pillow case. The cerebrospinal fluid (CSF) forms a yellow ring around the blood in the center of cotton cloth. This test has a limited usefulness, however, because research has found that saliva and saline also cause the same result.

142.

A. Oxygen is administered during the primary assessment. Because the patient is complaining of shortness of breath, applying oxygen is appropriate. The baseline vital signs will be assessed during the secondary assessment. A patient who is complaining of shortness of breath or one who displays signs of respiratory distress rarely tolerates being placed in a supine position. These patients typically are more comfortable in an upright position.

143.

D. The gurgling sound indicates that the patient has blood, vomitus, secretions, or some other substance in the airway. This requires immediate suction. Also, the patient has a respiratory rate of only six breaths per minute, which indicates inadequate breathing. After clearing the airway, positive pressure ventilation must be initiated.

144.

C. The respiratory rate of a newborn can be between 40 to 60 breaths per minute. As the infant grows older, the respiratory rate declines. Once the child reaches adolescence, the respiratory rate is close to that of an adult.

145.

B. A pulse oximeter is a very useful tool to indicate hypoxia in a patient. A real concern is a low pulse oximeter reading that persists after the application of a nonrebreather mask at 15 lpm. In this case, the patient is on a nonrebreather mask and his pulse oximetry (SpO_2) is still at 93 percent. With supplemental oxygen (especially a nonrebreather mask at 15 lpm), you would expect an SpO_2 reading near 100 percent. If the oxygen were removed from this patient, you would speculate that the SpO_2 reading would dip extremely low, indicating hypoxia. The patient's complaint of dyspnea does not correlate directly to the level of hypoxia. The skin is a better indicator of perfusion status, not hypoxia, even though you would expect to see cyanosis to the skin, which could be a late sign. The retractions and accessory muscle use are great indicators of respiratory distress and respiratory muscle work; however, these do not measure the level of hypoxia. You could assume that the patient in respiratory distress is hypoxic; however, other physical signs such as an altered mental status, head bobbing, agitation, and confusion are better indicators.

146.

C. Because the patient is responsive, the next step is to gather a SAMPLE history and then perform a focused physical exam during which you examine the abdomen and other related body systems. You should have already determined the level of responsiveness during the primary assessment. Also, it appears the patient is continuing to complain, indicating that his mental status has not changed. A rapid medical exam would be performed if the patient were unresponsive or had an altered mental status.

147.
C. The skin is the best indicator of the patient's perfusion status. During the primary assessment, you are trying to identify a life threat to the circulation.

148.
C. Fractured ribs are not considered possible life threats. If two or more ribs were fractured in two or more places creating a flail segment, this would be considered a life threatening injury. However, simple rib fractures are not life threatening unless they lacerate the lung or another underlying organ. A large laceration with oozing blood is not a life threat. If the bleeding were a steady flow or spurting, it would be considered a life threat. An angulated humerus is not a life threat unless associated with major bleeding. An open wound to the posterior thorax can lead to a significant amount of air trapped in the pleural space, causing the lung to collapse and would lead to a compromise in gas exchange and hypoxia.

149.
A. The patient's airway is open, the breathing is adequate, and his pulse is present; therefore, no airway ventilation intervention is necessary. However, his SpO2 reading is only 93%; therefore, you should initiate oxygen administration and perform a rapid medical assessment. Apply a nasal cannula at 2 to 4 lpm and continue to titrate the liter flow up until the SpO2 reaches 94% or greater. Spinal stabilization is not needed because no mechanism of trauma indicates a possible spine injury. The breathing is adequate; therefore, there is no need for bag-valve-mask ventilation. The vital signs will be taken as part of the rapid medical assessment. No transport should be conducted until after the assessment is completed.

150.
C. The skin is warm, dry, and normal in color. This indicates good tissue perfusion. Hypovolemic shock would result in poor tissue perfusion in which the skin would be pale, cool, and clammy. Hypoxia and inadequate delivery of hemoglobin would cause cyanosis.

151.
C. The unresponsive medical patient should be placed in a left lateral recumbent position, which is also known as the *coma* or *recovery position.* It is used to allow secretions and vomit to drain from the mouth and airway.

152.
D. Pain is a subjective complaint. You cannot assess and objectively determine whether the pain really exists or not. Some signs, such as a facial grimace, can tell you the severity of pain.

153.
D. The first priority is to determine whether the scene is safe. The best person at a building collapse to determine this is the engineer.

154.
C. Once the scene has been cleared of hazards, you should approach the patient, apply manual spinal stabilization, quickly assess the posterior thorax, and logroll the patient into a supine position.

155.
B. The primary assessment and rapid trauma and medical assessment are performed to identify and manage life-threatening injuries or conditions. The detailed secondary assessment is conducted to identify other nonlife-threatening injuries. Find life threats during the detailed physical exam, depends on indicates that you did not conduct a proper rapid trauma assessment. The detailed physical exam is the time available and the patient's condition. The means, that if you do not have the time or if the patient condition does not allow you to perform the detailed physical exam, it is acceptable not to perform it.

156.
A. Crackles, also know as *rales,* are be heard when the terminal bronchiole and alveoli collapse and re-expand with a breath. Wheezing indicates constricted bronchioles. Rhonchi is a

snoring type of sound that is heard when mucous collects in the larger airways. A pleural friction rub is a leathery creak sound heard on inhalation and exhalation.

157.
C. A patient who is found in a fetal position is most likely suffering from severe abdominal pain. The fetal position relieves some of the tension of the abdominal wall muscles and places less pressure on the underlying organs. Appendicitis can produce severe abdominal pain.

158.
A. This technique is assessing the consensual reflex, which causes both pupils to respond simultaneously to light even though it was shined in only one eye.

159.
C. Because the patient has an altered mental status, you must treat him under implied consent. It is best to have law enforcement present to assist and witness the restraint process. Do not restrain the patient in a prone position because doing so could interfere with his airway and impede his ventilation.

160.
D. A car on its roof is considered an unstable vehicle. The car could collapse under the weight, thus making it unsafe. The fire department must stabilize the vehicle prior to your entry.

161.
A. A patient who has suffered a blow to the face, nose, or area around the eye could have suffered a fracture to the bone on the bottom portion of the orbit under the eye (infraorbital). One sign of this type of fracture is the patient's a upward gaze of both eyes (conjugate gaze).

162.
A. An unresponsive patient with a fixed and dilated pupil following trauma to his head is most likely suffering from a brain injury with compression and herniation of brain tissue. A patient who is responsive and has a fixed and dilated pupil is not suffering from herniation of the brain but more likely an injury to the eye itself or an injury to the third cranial nerve.

163.
B. The brain controls function on the same side of the body above the level of the medulla at around the upper lip and on the opposite side of the body below the upper lip. An injury to the left side of the brain affects the left pupil and right extremities.

164.
A. Priapism is a persistent erection of the penis that may be a sign of spinal cord injury. Priapism can also be caused by use of some drugs or medical conditions such as sickle cell disease, malaria, or tumors.

165.
A. A rigid and tender abdomen is a sign of bleeding within the abdominal cavity (intra-abdominal bleeding). Pale, cool, and clammy skin and weak rapid radial pulses indicate poor perfusion.

166.
B. The abdominal cavity is covered by a peritoneal lining. Blood leaking into the peritoneal cavity irritates the lining. The irritation causes abdominal pain, tenderness on palpation, and abdominal wall guarding and rigidity.

167.
B. *Palliation* refers to any relief or alleviation of the symptom. Palliation of the breathing difficulty in this patient is achieved by putting him in an upright position.

168.
C. Tenderness and pain on palpation of the symphysis pubis usually indicates a pelvic fracture. When you assess the pelvis in a patient who

complained of pain prior to palpation, do not palpate. If the patient has no such complaint, press down and then inward on the anterior iliac crest, assessing for a pain response, instability, and crepitus. You should then apply pressure to the symphysis pubis.

169.
C. A patient with abdominal discomfort and pelvic pain can be suffering from a pelvic fracture and intra-abdominal bleeding. This patient is considered unstable; therefore, you should assess the vital signs every five minutes.

170.
B. Because the jugular vein drains into the superior vena cava that empties into the right atrium, a patient suffering from right-side heart failure is likely suffering from jugular venous distention.

171.
C. Assessing the ears and nose in a patient with chest pain is the least relevant. The oral mucosa could provide information about the oxygenation status. The breath sounds are important to assess for abnormal sounds or absence of breath sounds. The pedal pulses provide information about the perfusion status.

172.
B. To ensure that you have properly transferred the care of the patient to the emergency department, you must provide an oral report to medical personnel who are of equal or higher level of training than yourself. Until that official transfer of care is done, you must remain with the patient even in the emergency department.

173.
C. A deformed steering wheel in a rear-end collision indicates a significant mechanism of injury. A fall of less than twice the patient's height is not considered to be a significant mechanism of trauma. A fall of *more than* twice the patient's

height is considered a significant mechanism of injury. A gunshot wound to the lower leg is not considered significant because it lacks the potential to injure major organs. Be aware of major bleeding associated with the gunshot wound that can make it an immediate life threat. An auto crash of 20 miles per hour is considered a low-velocity crash that can still produce injury, sometimes significant, but this likelihood is less than that of a high-velocity crash.

174.
C. A component of the scene size-up is to determine the number of patients and call for additional resources. If several patients are found on entering the scene, you should call for additional resources at that time.

175.
B. Because the laceration of the leg could be a wound with major bleeding, immediately expose the extremity and inspect the wound. Once the bleeding has been controlled, continue the primary assessment.

176.
A. A 78-year-old patient who cannot remember his name has an altered mental status. Any patient with an altered mental status is considered to be a priority.

177.
B. Clear fluid coming from the nose, ears, or mouth following trauma to the head can be cerebrospinal fluid (CSF). CSF leakage usually is found when the patient has suffered a skull fracture. Test with the glucometer to determine whether the fluid is CSF. CSF contains glucose, even though the amount is much less than whole or capillary blood. Nasal secretions do not contain glucose.

178.
B. Assessing a blood pressure in children less than three years of age is difficult. It is more important to rely on peripheral and central pulses

and the skin signs to determine perfusion status. It is difficult to assess the orientation in a two-year-old patient. The reddened sclera does not apply to a dehydrated patient.

179.
B. A patient with an altered mental status may not be able to control his own airway. Therefore, it is important that you carefully assess and monitor the airway of any patient with an altered mental status.

180.
C. Scene safety is your first concern. Until the scene is determined to be safe, you should remain in the ambulance.

181.
B. During exhalation, the chest wall is moving inward. A segment that moves opposite or outward when the remainder of the chest is moving inward is considered to be moving in a paradoxical motion, which indicates a flail segment.

182.
D. *Stridor* is a high-pitched sound produced from air rushing past a partial obstruction at the level of the larynx. It is commonly produced by swelling in the larynx.

183.
D. Because the patient is talking when you arrive at her side, you have already determined that she is alert, her airway is patent, and her breathing is adequate. The next step in the primary assessment is to assess the pulse and skin.

184.
B. A patient with hot, dry skin can be suffering from a heat-related emergency such as heat stroke. This is a dire emergency that requires rapid treatment and transport. Shock and heart attack normally produce cool and diaphoretic skin. A stroke usually presents with no significant skin findings.

185.
D. The patient's mental status is the key to whether to perform the rapid medical assessment or SAMPLE history first. If the patient is unable to respond appropriately to your questions, you should proceed with the rapid medical assessment.

186.
D. Any female patient in child-bearing years complaining of abdominal pain should be questioned about her menstrual period. You need to determine whether she has missed one, any abnormal discharge has occurred, bleeding has occurred between the period, or the period was excessively heavy. This can provide a clue to whether the condition could be related to a reproductive organ injury or disorder.

187.
C. The patient has tachycardia. A heart rate of more than 100 beats per minute in an adult patient is considered to be tachycardia. A narrow pulse pressure occurs when the difference between the systolic and diastolic blood pressure is less than 30 mmHg. *Tachypnea* is a respiratory rate that is more than 20 per minute in the adult. *Hypertension* is defined as a systolic blood pressure of more than 160 mmHg and a diastolic of more than 90 mmHg.

188.
D. Apply an occlusive dressing to any wound to the thorax. Regardless of whether the wound is anterior, lateral, or posterior, it can still be a sucking chest wound. This type of wound could easily produce a tension pneumothorax.

189.
B. The medical term for *swelling* is *edema*. *Erythema* is redness; *ecchymosis* means discoloration of a black and blue tint; and a *contusion* is a bruise.

190.
B. Once the posterior neck or cervical region has been palpated, it is necessary to apply the cervical spinal immobilization collar. Once the collar has been applied, manual spinal stabilization must still be maintained until the patient is fully immobilized to the backboard.

191.
B. Because aspiration interferes with gas exchange in the alveoli and produces hypoxia, cyanosis can occur.

192.
D. Even if the patient refuses, attempt to persuade her to allow you to assess her injury. It is important to be sure that you inform the patient of the possible consequences of the possible injuries.

193.
C. A systemic allergic reaction, also known as *anaphylaxis,* causes the bronchioles to constrict and become inflamed on the internal surface. This increase in airway resistance produces wheezing when air rushes through.

194.
C. Palliation or alleviation is reported when a medication, position, activity, or lack of activity reduces the severity of the symptom or eliminates it.

195.
D. Approximately 50 percent of the patients who suffer a tonic-clonic seizure bite the tongue. If you arrive on the scene of a patient who has a laceration to the tongue, you should suspect a possible seizure.

196.
D. *Subcutaneous emphysema* is air trapped under the skin. It indicates a leak in the respiratory tract lung or the esophagus. It could be easier to feel the bubble packaging texture than to see the bloated look of the skin when performing your assessment. In the seated patient, the air normally travels upward to the upper chest, neck, and face.

197.
D. A detailed physical exam may be skipped. It is designed to identify injuries that are not life threatening; therefore, it is more important to focus on life threats than to assess for injuries that are not life threatening.

198.
D. Because the heart is compressed in the mediastinum during tension pneumothorax, the cardiac output is reduced and the systolic blood pressure decreased. The pulse pressure becomes narrowed when the systolic and diastolic blood pressure readings become closer together.

199.
B. All patients, regardless of how serious or minor the extent of the injury or illness, must have an primary assessment.

200.
C. You should immediately repeat the primary assessment to determine whether her airway is still patent and her breathing is still adequate and to reassess her pulse and skin. You should then repeat the assessment of the abdomen and obtain another set of vital signs.

201.
A. The purpose of the rapid trauma assessment is to identify and manage life threats to the patient. All other injuries that are not life threats are identified and managed during the detailed physical exam.

202.
C. The fact that a patient says a few words and then must gasp for a breath is a good indication that he is having difficulty breathing. A crying patient or one who talks with a completely normal

speech pattern typically is not having a difficult time breathing.

203.

B. A fall from the roof of a house would indicate a spinal injury. Therefore, it is necessary to take manual spinal stabilization prior to making the primary assessment.

204.

D. The patient has inadequate respirations. Because the patient is not responding to painful stimuli, you can insert an oropharyngeal airway to facilitate the ventilation.

205.

B. *Tenderness* is pain on palpation. *Rigidity* is an involuntary abdominal muscle contraction. *Guarding* is voluntary abdominal muscle contraction. *Pain* is a patient complaint that occurs without any palpation or manipulation of the area.

4 Medical/Gynecology/Obstetrics

DIRECTIONS Each of the questions or incomplete statements below is followed by suggested answers or completions. Select the **one answer** that is best in each case.

General Pharmacology

1. A medication that can be administered by an EMT that is carried on the ambulance is:
   A. epinephrine.
   B. oral glucose.
   C. beta 2 inhaler.
   D. nitroglycerin.

2. EMTs can assist with administration of which of the following medications?
   A. intravenous epinephrine
   B. valium by mouth
   C. intramuscular glucagon
   D. beta 2 metered dose inhalers

3. Which of the following is a medication that the EMT can assist the patient in taking during a respiratory emergency?
   A. Albuterol
   B. Decadron
   C. Atrovent
   D. Benadryl

4. The drug action of Actidose and SuperChar is to:
   A. increase the blood glucose level in the hypoglycemic patient.
   B. bind with certain poisons to prevent further absorption.
   C. relax the coronary arteries in patients having chest pain.
   D. dilate the bronchioles in the asthma patient.

5. The generic name(s) for Alupent is:
   A. albuterol.
   B. isoetharine.
   C. metaproterenol.
   D. diphenhydramine.

6. You are called to the scene for an unknown medical emergency. Upon arrival, you find a 43-year-old female patient sitting in a tripod position at the kitchen table. She complains that she "can't breathe" and appears to be in significant respiratory distress. You find her respirations are 29 per minute and labored. Her radial pulse is 124/minute. Her skin is pale, cool, and clammy. Her pulse oximeter reading is 86 percent. You hear wheezing in all lung fields upon auscultating her lungs. Which medication prescribed to her would you administer?
   A. Daizepam
   B. Digoxin
   C. Methylprednisolone
   D. Salmeterol xinafoate

7. If you are unsure about a generic name on a medication, you should:
   A. ask the patient whether the generic name is the same as the trade name with which you are familiar.
   B. administer the drug immediately because any delay in administration could harm the patient.
   C. contact medical direction and ask for information.
   D. attempt to find the drug insert information.

8. The generic name of a medication is:
   A. used when the drug is approved by the FDA.
   B. similar to the chemical name of the medication.
   C. the name is listed in the U.S. Pharmacopoeia.
   D. all of the above

9. Which of the following is an approved medication carried on an EMT ambulance?
   A. oral glutose
   B. Bronkosol
   C. albuterol
   D. nitrostat

10. A drug that contains both strong alpha and beta properties is:
    A. metaproterenol.
    B. epinephrine.
    C. albuterol.
    D. Inderal.

11. After administering a medication you should:
    A. repeat the dose until the desired effect has been achieved.
    B. ask the patient if he feels that the medication is working.
    C. reassess the patient to determine whether the medication was effective.
    D. ask the patient if he feels that it is becoming harder to breathe.

12. Which of the following drug routes of administration is *incorrectly* paired?
    A. sublingual—nitroglycerin spray under the tongue
    B. oral—swallowing a nitroglycerin tablet
    C. inhalation—topical deposition of beta$_2$ drugs on bronchial smooth muscle
    D. injection—intramuscular administration of epinephrine

Respiratory Emergencies

13. Which anatomical structure is found outside the respiratory tract?
    A. bronchi
    B. alveoli
    C. diaphragm
    D. carina

14. Which of the following is a function of the nose and nasopharynx?
    A. to prevent the aspiration of substances into the trachea
    B. to block the oropharynx when swallowing
    C. to trap air when speaking
    D. to humidify inspired air

15. Which structure is responsible for directing food to the esophagus and air into the trachea?
    A. hypopharynx
    B. epiglottis
    C. carina
    D. cricoid cartilage

16. Which muscle(s) contributes 60 percent to 75 percent of the effort to breathe?
    A. external intercostal muscles
    B. internal intercostal muscles
    C. diaphragm
    D. pectoralis major

17. When an adult patient initially becomes hypoxic, you would expect the heart rate to:
    A. increase due to sympathetic discharge.
    B. decrease due to parasympathetic discharge.
    C. increase due to parasympathetic discharge.
    D. decrease due to sympathetic discharge.

18. An early sign of hypoxia in the adult, child, and infant is:
    A. unresponsiveness.
    B. cyanosis.
    C. bradycardia.
    D. restlessness.

19. To determine whether the patient is breathing adequately, you must assess the:
    A. tidal volume and breath sounds.
    B. breath sounds bilaterally.
    C. respiratory rate and tidal volume.
    D. heart rate and chest rise and fall.

20. Which is a sign of adequate ventilation?
    A. The bluish discoloration to the oral mucosa turns gray.
    B. The patient appears relaxed, is sleeping, and no longer resists the ventilation.
    C. Bilateral chest rise and fall occurs with each ventilation.
    D. Upward movement of the abdomen occurs with each ventilation.

21. The proportionate size of the tongue in an infant when compared with that of an adult is:
    A. smaller.
    B. larger.
    C. equal in size.
    D. extremely small.

22. What is the narrowest portion of the upper airway in infants and children under ten years of age?
    A. posterior oral pharynx
    B. epiglottic opening
    C. glottic opening
    D. cricoid ring

23. You arrive on the scene to find a frantic mother screaming that her daughter cannot breathe. The infant is making high-pitched sounds on inspiration, has good color, is alert, and is gasping for air. You suspect what problem?
    A. acute bronchitis
    B. partial airway obstruction
    C. asthma attack
    D. complete airway obstruction

24. When treating an adult patient with a partial airway obstruction as compared to a complete airway obstruction, the following assessment or treatment applies:
    A. In a complete obstruction, provide oxygen by nonrebreather mask but give no oxygen in a partial obstruction.
    B. In a partial obstruction, attempt to view the obstruction, but in a complete obstruction do not perform visualization.
    C. In a partial obstruction, instruct the patient to cough, but in a complete obstruction, deliver abdominal thrusts.
    D. The priority is placed on removing the obstruction in the partial obstruction, but immediate transport is the key management for a complete obstruction.

25. A common sign indicating a complete airway obstruction is that:
    A. the patient does not cry or talk.
    B. a decreased amount of air is heard and felt on exhalation.
    C. the patient coughs forcefully.
    D. breath sounds decrease bilaterally.

26. During the mechanical process of inhalation, the:
    A. diaphragm and intercostal muscles contract.
    B. diaphragm contracts, and the intercostal muscles relax.
    C. diaphragm relaxes, and the intercostal muscles contract.
    D. diaphragm and the intercostal muscles relax.

27. The process of exchanging oxygen and carbon dioxide at the cell is known as:
    A. oxygenation.
    B. ventilation.

C. inspiration.

D. respiration.

28. The structure that has a common opening for the respiratory tract and the digestive system is the:

    A. larynx.

    B. esophagus.

    C. trachea.

    D. pharynx.

29. A common cause of upper airway obstruction in a young child is flexion of the head commonly caused by:

    A. the child's head being proportionately smaller than the rest of the body.

    B. the trachea being underdeveloped.

    C. the child's tongue being so big it forces the forward flexion.

    D. the child's head being disproportionately larger than the rest of the body.

30. What anatomic structure covers the outer portion of the lung?

    A. parietal peritoneum

    B. bronchiole smooth muscle

    C. pericardial sac

    D. visceral pleura

31. You are managing a patient in respiratory distress who is wheezing. A family member brings you a metered-dose inhaler. You can assist the patient with its administration only if:

    A. the wheezing is in one lung field.

    B. the dose is printed on the label.

    C. the medication does not expire for more than six months.

    D. it is prescribed to the patient.

32. What are the two major anatomical divisions of the pharynx?

    A. larynx and trachea

    B. larynx and oropharynx

C. larynx and nasopharynx

D. oropharynx and nasopharynx

33. The larynx is commonly referred to as the:

    A. windpipe.

    B. esophagus.

    C. voice box.

    D. master gland.

34. You are called to a residence for a man who is having difficulty breathing. While you are assessing the patient, his wife hands you the telephone stating it is the family doctor. The doctor identifies himself and orders you to administer two puffs of the wife's metered-dose inhaler because it sounds as if the husband is suffering from the same type of asthma attacks his wife does. You should:

    A. follow the order because a physician gave it.

    B. advise the physician that you will follow his orders only if he meets you at the emergency room and signs your run report.

    C. explain to the physician that it is against your protocol to help administer the medication because it is not prescribed for your patient.

    D. tell the physician you can perform the order if he writes a prescription for the medication for your patient.

35. Before consulting with medical direction for an order to administer a medication, the EMT should:

    A. check the package insert in the medication to verify that it is the right drug.

    B. check a drug source for the correct dose to be administered to the patient.

    C. call for an advanced life support unit in case the patient deteriorates.

    D. assess the patient to identify and manage life threats.

36. You are administering oxygen to a patient who is complaining of shortness of breath. The initial auscultation of the lungs revealed inspiratory and expiratory wheezing in all lung fields. After administering the oxygen, you reassess the patient and find decreased wheezing in all lung fields and diminished breath sounds bilaterally. This is an indication that:
    A. the oxygen therapy is effective because the wheezing is decreasing.
    B. the bronchoconstriction is worsening and the patient is deteriorating.
    C. bronchodilation is occurring in the terminal bronchioles, and the patient should improve.
    D. the patient is relaxing and no longer working as hard to breathe.

37. A sign of adequate ventilation is:
    A. the resistance increases when squeezing the bag of the bag-valve mask.
    B. the patient begins to push the mask away from his face.
    C. the heart rate increases from 98 to 118 beats per minute.
    D. the oropharyngeal airway remains seated on the teeth.

38. _____ indicates an upper airway partial obstruction while _____ indicates a lower airway obstruction.
    A. Wheezing, stridor
    B. Wheezing, crackles or rales
    C. Stridor, wheezing
    D. Stridor, crackles or rales

39. Asthma is a(n) _____ airway disease and epiglottitis is a(n) _____ airway disease.
    A. upper, lower
    B. lower, upper
    C. upper, upper
    D. lower, lower

40. A tripod position is most often a presenting sign in a patient who is experiencing:
    A. respiratory distress.
    B. hypoglycemia.
    C. a stroke.
    D. a heat emergency.

41. The term used to describe the condition of a patient who is no longer breathing is:
    A. dyspnea.
    B. bradypnea.
    C. tachypnea.
    D. apnea.

42. Choose the sign or symptom that best indicates severe respiratory distress.
    A. A patient complains of chest pain when walking up steps.
    B. A patient has a bluish-gray skin color around the nose and mouth.
    C. A ten-year-old is breathing 30 times each minute.
    D. A four-month-old's abdomen rises with each inhalation.

43. Stridor upon inhalation is an indication of a:
    A. traumatic flail segment.
    B. tension pneumothorax.
    C. sucking chest wound.
    D. partial airway obstruction.

44. A late sign of respiratory failure in an infant or young child is:
    A. tachycardia.
    B. nasal flaring.
    C. hypotension.
    D. retractions.

45. You are assessing a 56-year-old male patient whom you suspect has suffered a head injury because of his altered mental status. The patient responds to painful stimuli by moaning. His airway is clear and he has a respiratory rate of 16/minute with shallow chest rise. You should immediately:
    A. administer oxygen via a nonrebreather mask.
    B. begin bag-valve-mask ventilation.
    C. insert an nasopharyngeal airway.
    D. place the patient in the lateral recumbent position.

46. You are treating a 67-year-old female patient with a history of shortness of breath due to pneumonia. Her vital signs are blood pressure 178/84 mmHg; respiration, 22 with good chest rise; P, 108 beats/minute; and SpO_2, 94 percent. You should:
    A. immediately begin bag-valve-mask ventilation.
    B. administer oxygen via a nasal cannula at 2 lpm.
    C. seek permission to administer a beta 2 agonist.
    D. contact medical direction before administering oxygen.

47. A sign of respiratory failure in an infant is:
    A. loss of muscle tone (limp appearance).
    B. cyanosis around the mouth and nose.
    C. an increasing heart rate.
    D. prolonged exhalation.

48. You are treating an apprehensive child who is experiencing difficulty breathing. The child will not tolerate the nonrebreather mask and continuously removes it from his face. You should:
    A. do nothing because the child cannot be in distress if he can resist treatment.
    B. have a parent hold the mask near the child's face to deliver the oxygen.

    C. speak to the child calmly while holding the mask over his mouth and nose.
    D. place the child on a nasal cannula at 2 lpm and have him breathe only through his nose.

49. You are treating a four-year-old male who complains of a bad sore throat. His voice is hoarse when he speaks with you. He says only a couple of words with each answer and appears very still. The child is sitting upright and leaning forward, has his neck jutted out, and is drooling. He is breathing 36 time per minute with a decreased tidal volume. He has a fever. You should:
    A. insert an oropharyngeal airway and begin bag-valve-mask ventilation.
    B. perform a finger sweep to remove a suspected foreign object.
    C. administer oxygen via a nonrebreather mask and begin immediate transport.
    D. suction any secretions from the oropharynx with a hard suction catheter.

50. The aerosolized medication contained within the metered-dose inhaler has what action?
    A. beta agonist that relaxes the bronchiole smooth muscle
    B. beta agonist that contracts the tracheal smooth muscle
    C. alpha agonist that relaxes the bronchiole smooth muscle
    D. alpha agonist that contracts the tracheal smooth muscle

51. A contraindication to the administration of a bronchodilator by metered-dose inhaler is:
    A. a history of bronchoconstriction.
    B. a patient who does not respond to verbal stimuli.
    C. a patient who has already taken one dose of the medication.
    D. wheezing in all lung fields upon auscultation.

52. You are preparing to assist the patient with the administration of her metered-dose inhaler. You have already obtained an order from medical direction and confirmed the medication dose, expiration date, and route. When coaching the patient, what should you instruct her to do immediately after she inhales the medication?
   A. Rapidly exhale and then hold her breath for approximately 5 seconds.
   B. Cough forcefully and continuously as she exhales the medication.
   C. Attempt to hold her breath for up to 10 seconds and breathe out through pursed lips.
   D. Take several rapid and deep breaths to replenish the oxygen used during the procedure.

53. Which of the following is inappropriate for the EMT to administer due to its delayed action?
   A. Ventolin
   B. Alupent
   C. isoetharine
   D. ipratropium bromide (Atrovent®)

54. After assisting your patient with a metered-dose inhaler, he experiences tachycardia and nervousness. Which of the following is true regarding this finding?
   A. These are common side effects of the drug.
   B. The patient has overdosed on the medication.
   C. These occurred because the medication dose was incorrect.
   D. The patient is hypersensitive to the drug.

55. You are treating a four-year-old patient who complains of a sore throat and fever. The mother states that the child has had a cold for about a week and it seems to get worse at night. During the day, the child is still active; however, he has had a hoarse voice for three to four days. When he seems to be worse, he has a harsh, metallic or barking seal cough. His vital signs are blood pressure, 92/62 mmHg; heart rate, 104 beats/minute; respiration, 28; and pulse oximeter reading, 94 percent on room air. You suspect the patient most likely has:
   A. croup.
   B. epiglottitis.
   C. asthma.
   D. a foreign body obstruction.

56. Which of the following signs and symptoms indicate lower airway disease in a child?
   A. audible wheezes and diminished breath sounds
   B. cough that produces a sound like a barking seal
   C. fever, stridorous airway sounds, drooling
   D. sudden onset of stridorous airway sounds

57. You are assessing a six-year-old child who presents with shortness of breath and wheezing. The patient is prescribed Proventil® by metered-dose inhaler. You suspect that the patient has a history of:
   A. emphysema.
   B. epiglottitis.
   C. asthma.
   D. croup.

Cardiovascular Emergenices

58. Blood is ejected from the right atrium into the:
   A. right ventricle.
   B. left ventricle.
   C. pulmonary arteries.
   D. pulmonary veins.

59. The exchange of oxygen, carbon dioxide, and other vital nutrients takes place between the blood and the cells in the:
    A. pulmonary arteries.
    B. capillaries.
    C. arterioles.
    D. pulmonary veins.

60. The pressure of blood in the two separate sides of the heart can be described as:
    A. low pressure in the left myocardium and high pressure in the right myocardium.
    B. high pressure in the right myocardium and high pressure in the left myocardium.
    C. low pressure in the right myocardium and high pressure in the left myocardium.
    D. low pressure in the right myocardium and low pressure in the left myocardium.

61. The automated external defibrillator should be applied to which patient?
    A. a 6-month-old child with minimal chest wall movement and a respiratory rate of 62 per minute
    B. a 17-year-old drug overdose patient with a heart rate of 32 beats/minute
    C. a 55-year-old patient who was complaining of chest pain and is now unresponsive
    D. a 43-year-old patient with a cardiac pacemaker who collapsed and is pulseless and with a gasping type breath

62. The best position to transport the patient complaining of shortness of breath is with the patient:
    A. supine, allowing for access to the airway.
    B. supine with the feet elevated to reduce the edema of the ankles.
    C. in a Fowler's position.
    D. in a lateral recumbent position.

63. What is the most common presenting rhythm within the first 8 minutes after a patient goes into cardiac arrest?
    A. asystole
    B. ventricular tachycardia
    C. ventricular fibrillation
    D. pulseless electrical activity

64. The most effective treatment to terminate ventricular fibrillation is:
    A. cardiopulmonary resuscitation.
    B. hyperventilation.
    C. defibrillation.
    D. drug therapy.

65. Why should advanced life support (ALS) be requested in a cardiac arrest when the EMT is able to defibrillate the patient?
    A. The patient can be transferred to the ALS unit and place the basic unit back into service more quickly.
    B. Prehospital ALS is integral in the chain of survival and needs to be activated quickly to allow for speedier definitive care.
    C. The fee for the ALS unit is higher and generates more revenue.
    D. The ALS unit carries a monitor/ defibrillator in case the automated external defibrillator malfunctions.

66. The major difference between a semiautomatic and automatic defibrillator is that:
    A. the semiautomatic defibrillator provides a better "picture" of the heart.
    B. the automatic defibrillator requires more operator involvement.
    C. the automatic defibrillator requires constant contact with the patient during defibrillation.
    D. the semiautomatic defibrillator requires the operator to push a button to deliver a shock.

67. How many initial defibrillations should be delivered to a patient in cardiac arrest?
    A. one set of three defibrillations
    B. two defibrillations
    C. three defibrillations with 1 minute of CPR between each set of three
    D. one defibrillation

68. You are treating a patient complaining of chest pain when he suddenly collapses. You verify that he is unresponsive, pulseless, and apneic. Your first immediate action is to:
    A. perform five cycles of CPR, attach the defibrillator, and shock if advised.
    B. deliver a precordial thump and deliver ten cycles of CPR.
    C. perform CPR until the advanced life support unit arrives to perform manual defibrillation.
    D. immediately attach the defibrillator and shock if advised.

69. A case review is beneficial after use of the automated external defibrillator (AED) to:
    A. penalize crews who have poor response times.
    B. determine whether the AED is appropriately delivering shocks.
    C. improve the coordination of advanced life support responding units in the system.
    D. determine whether the EMT should manually analyze the rhythm before defibrillation.

70. You respond to the scene and find a patient in cardiac arrest. The first shock from the automated external defibrillator should be delivered:
    A. within 60 seconds after arriving at the patient's side.
    B. following five cycles of CPR.
    C. after delivering two ventilations by bag-valve-mask unit.
    D. following 5 minutes of CPR.

71. You are treating a cardiac arrest patient and have just delivered the first defibrillation to the patient using the automated external defibrillator. Your next immediate action is to:
    A. resume chest compressions and continue CPR for five cycles.
    B. deliver two breaths and resume chest compressions.
    C. deliver a second defibrillation ar 300 joules or the biphasic equivalent.
    D. assess the pulse and breathing followed by another defibrillation.

72. The most common cause of automated external defibrillator failure is:
    A. electronic malfunction.
    B. improper placement of the pads.
    C. patient artifact.
    D. a weak or dead battery.

73. The operator checklist of the automated external defibrillator (AED) should be completed:
    A. once per month.
    B. once per week.
    C. at the beginning of each shift or at least once daily.
    D. only when the AED itself identifies the malfunction.

74. To be most effective in converting ventricular fibrillation into a perfusing rhythm, when should defibrillation be performed following an unwitnessed cardiac arrest?
    A. immediately upon arrival at the scene
    B. after the delivery of two breaths and one cycle of CPR
    C. after advanced life support has arrived and administered medications to the patient
    D. following five cycles of CPR

75. If proper bystander CPR is being performed, defibrillation is most successful in converting the patient with an intact neurologic status for up to how many minutes after the onset of cardiac arrest?
    A. 5 minutes
    B. 8 minutes
    C. 10 minutes
    D. 12 minutes

76. After the delivery of the first defibrillation, CPR should be performed for:
    A. 1 minute followed by another defibrillation.
    B. 5 minutes followed by analysis of the rhythm.
    C. until the automated external defibrillator indicates a shock is advised.
    D. five cycles prior to analyzing the rhythm.

77. After delivering a defibrillation, your next immediate action is to:
    A. check the carotid pulse.
    B. deliver another defibrillation.
    C. begin chest compressions.
    D. deliver two ventilations.

78. To which patient is it most appropriate to attach an automated external defibrillator?
    A. an unresponsive patient who has cyanosis to the face
    B. a apneic patient who has a weak carotid pulse
    C. an unresponsive hypoglycemic patient who has no carotid pulse
    D. a patient with a severe head injury who is in cardiac arrest

79. While you are preparing the automated external defibrillator to defibrillate the cardiac arrest patient, your partner should be:
    A. preparing a backboard and the cot for rapid transport.
    B. performing five cycles of CPR.
    C. gathering a medical history from family or bystanders.
    D. performing ventilation only with the bag-valve-mask device.

80. What are the initial steps for a single rescuer to take to manage an unwitnessed cardiac arrest patient?
    A. Immediately apply the automated external defibrillator and analyze the patient rhythm.
    B. Do CPR for 1 minute, apply the automated external defibrillator, and analyze the rhythm.
    C. Oxygenate the patient with positive pressure ventilation only for 1 minute, apply the automated external defibrillator, and analyze the rhythm.
    D. Do five cycles of CPR, apply the automated external defibrillator, and analyze the rhythm.

81. After successfully defibrillating your patient, you are en route to rendezvous with advanced life support backup. You have applied oxygen and left the automated external defibrillator on the patient. The patient suddenly becomes pulseless and apneic. You should?
    A. analyze the cardiac rhythm
    B. remove the AED so no additional shocks are delivered
    C. begin bag-valve-mask ventilation
    D. start five cycles of CPR

82. You are transporting to the ambulance a patient who has been defibrillated three times before regaining a pulse. The patient suddenly becomes apneic, and the automated external defibrillator indicates that the patient is in a shockable rhythm. You should immediately:

    A. begin CPR and rapid transport.

    B. shock the patient once and begin CPR.

    C. deliver three stacked shocks.

    D. wait for the advanced life support unit to administer drugs before defibrillating again.

83. How often should you reassess the postresuscitation patient during transport?

    A. when the patient begins to experience chest pain

    B. once during a 20-minute transport

    C. at least every 5 minutes or whenever the patient's condition changes

    D. every 15 minutes if the patient's condition does not change

84. The fully automated external defibrillator differs from the semiautomatic external defibrillator in which of the following aspects?

    A. The fully automated external defibrillator will not discharge the machine while a rescuer is still in contact with the patient.

    B. The fully automated external defibrillator analyzes the rhythm and delivers the shock itself.

    C. The fully automated external defibrillator delivers the shocks at a higher joule setting.

    D. The fully automated external defibrillator delivers the stacked shocks at a slower rate.

85. Which of the following is the most critical element in successful defibrillation?

    A. number of EMS responders

    B. ability to secure an airway with an endotracheal tube

    C. ability to administer cardiac medications within the first minute following cardiac arrest

    D. time to defibrillation

86. You are working in a rural county as an EMT. You answer a call at a physician's office for a patient with chest pain. The physician informs you the patient is experiencing a myocardial infarction. The physician orders you to administer nitroglycerin every 5 minutes for the entire trip to the emergency department (approximately 30 minutes away). You are unable to contact the on-line medical direction to discuss what to do. As a prudent EMT, you should:

    A. transport the patient and follow the physician's orders.

    B. transport the patient and administer the nitroglycerin every 5 minutes only if the patient's systolic blood pressure remains above 90 mmHg.

    C. advise the physician that it is against your protocol and you cannot administer the nitroglycerin as he has ordered.

    D. call dispatch to send the advanced life support unit in the neighboring county to transport the patient and place your unit back in service.

87. You are treating a patient who is complaining of chest pain. You should place the patient in a:

    A. full Fowler's position.

    B. supine position.

    C. Trendelenburg position.

    D. position of comfort.

88. The batteries in the automated external defibrillator should be checked:

    A. monthly.

    B. daily.

    C. weekly.

    D. semiannually.

89. Any time the automated external defibrillator advises "No Shock," you should:
    A. stop and turn the machine off.
    B. disconnect its leads, leaving only the patches in place on the patient's chest.
    C. immediately begin chest compressions.
    D. reanalyze the rhythm to be sure the rhythm is nonshockable.

90. Which of the following is a contraindication for using the automated external defibrillator?
    A. a six-year-old child
    B. a five-month-old infant
    C. a patient with an implanted automatic cardiac defibrillator device
    D. a patient with an extremely weak and slow carotid pulse

91. Arrange the following steps in order for use of the automated external defibrillator in the unwitnessed cardiac arrest.
    1. Take body substance isolation precautions.
    2. Deliver shock.
    3. Perform five cycles of CPR.
    4. Attach the automated external defibrillator.
    5. Assess for responsiveness, breathing and pulse.

    A. 1, 4, 2, 5, 3
    B. 1, 5, 4, 2, 3
    C. 1, 5, 3, 4, 2
    D. 5, 1, 4, 2, 3

92. Before administering a second dose of nitroglycerin, you must:
    A. determine the blood pressure.
    B. attach the pulse oximeter.
    C. recheck the medication.
    D. inspect inside the patient's mouth.

93. The right side of the heart:
    A. receives blood from the arteries of the heart and pumps oxygenated blood to the left ventricle.
    B. receives oxygen-depleted blood from the veins of the body and pumps the blood to the peripheral tissues.
    C. receives oxygen-depleted blood from the arteries and pumps oxygenated blood to the left side of the heart.
    D. receives oxygen-depleted blood from the veins and pumps the oxygenated blood to the lungs.

94. You are treating a patient who complains of chest discomfort with no shortness of breath. The respiratory rate is 22/minute with a good volume. The SpO2 is 90%. You should administer oxygen by:
    A. nasal cannula at 6 lpm.
    B. nonrebreather mask at 15 lpm.
    C. nasal cannula at 2 lpm.
    D. nonrebreather mask at 6 lpm.

95. You are treating a 58-year-old male patient complaining of chest discomfort with shortness of breath that has lasted for more than 3 hours. The vital signs are blood pressure, 178/102 mmHg; heart rate, 108 beats/minute; respiration, 18 per minute with adequate chest rise; and pulse oximeter reading 96 percent. You should:
    A. administer a beta 2 agonist by metered-dose inhaler.
    B. place the patient in the Trendelenburg position.
    C. begin bag-valve-mask ventilation at 10 to 12 ventilation/minute.
    D. administer oxygen by nasal cannula.

96. You arrive on the scene and find an unrepsonsive 68-year-old patient who had been complaining of severe chest tightness prior to your arrival. The vital signs are blood pressure, 92/68 mmHg; heart rate, 36 beats/minute; respiration, 12/minute and shallow; and pulse oximeter reading, 84 percent. The skin is pale, cool, and clammy. You should immediately:
    A. place the patient in a lateral recumbent position.
    B. insert an oropharyngeal airway.
    C. apply a nonrebreather mask at 15 lpm.
    D. begin bag-valve-mask ventilation.

97. Patients who are diabetic and elderly can present with a:
    A. silent heart attack.
    B. muted heart attack.
    C. tranquil heart attack.
    D. quiet heart attack.

98. By what route is nitroglycerin spray administered?
    A. topical
    B. sublingual
    C. ingestion
    D. injection

99. In which of the following patient presentations is nitroglycerin contraindicated?
    A. 62-year-old, lightheaded, heart rate, 80/minute; blood pressure, 98/52 mmHg; and respiration, 20/minute
    B. 72-year-old who is very anxious, heart rate, 102/minute; blood pressure, 158/88 mmHg; and respirations, 26/minute
    C. 46-year-old who has taken two doses of nitroglycerin, heart rate, 110/minute; blood pressure, 142/68 mmHg; and respiration, 22/minute
    D. 86-year-old with an irregular heart rate of 86/minute, difficulty breathing at 38/minute, blood pressure at 186/80 mmHg

100. Which of the following is a common side effect of nitroglycerin?
    A. increase in systolic blood pressure
    B. tachycardia
    C. abdominal pain
    D. blurred vision

101. A 42-year-old male patient is complaining of a severe substernal chest discomfort, dyspnea, and nausea. You should next:
    A. assess the radial pulse and skin color, temperature, and condition.
    B. obtain a SAMPLE history from the patient or relatives at the scene.
    C. insert an oropharyngeal airway and begin bag-valve-mask ventilation.
    D. apply the automated external defibrillator and allow it to analyze the rhythm.

102. Which of the following is a link in the American Heart Association's chain of survival for patients with cardiac arrest?
    A. early diagnosis
    B. early cardiac pacing
    C. effective advanced life support
    D. early intravenous therapy

103. Which of the following statements is *incorrect* pertaining to ventricular fibrillation and defibrillation?
    A. Ventricular fibrillation is the most common initial rhythm in sudden cardiac arrest.
    B. Early electrical defibrillation is the most successful treatment for ventricular fibrillation.
    C. When CPR is performed, successful defibrillation time can be extended.
    D. Ventricular fibrillation lasts long periods of time before deteriorating to asystole.

104. If an advanced life support (paramedic) unit is not available to assist you after the initial defibrillation, you should:
    A. continue to defibrillate the patient until the rhythm changes to asystole.
    B. pronounce the patient dead.
    C. continue with CPR and defibrillation.
    D. remain on the scene and provide CPR only.

105. Which of the following represents the correct placement of monophasic defibrillator adhesive pads on a cardiac arrest patient?
    A. The (+) is placed below the xiphoid process below the sternum; the (−) is placed over the ribs at the right anterior axillary line.
    B. The (−) is placed below the xiphoid process below the sternum; the (+) is placed over the ribs at the right anterior axillary line.
    C. The (+) is placed on the right upper border of the sternum; the (−) is placed over the ribs at the left anterior axillary line.
    D. The (−) is placed on the right upper border of the sternum; the (+) is placed over the left lower ribs at the left anterior axillary line.

106. You have delivered the first shock using a semi-automated external defibrillator (AED). You should:
    A. immediately begin chest compressions.
    B. deliver a second shock.
    C. reposition the adhesive pads.
    D. check pulse and if it has not been regained, begin CPR immediately.

107. The major difference between a semiautomated external defibrillator and a fully automated external defibrillator is:
    A. the semiautomated one recognizes asystole and will deliver a shock.
    B. the semiautomated one is designed to be used on children and adults.
    C. the fully automated one delivers a shock without operation intervention when appropriate.
    D. the fully automated one can effectively analyze the rhythm during CPR.

108. Why must CPR be stopped while the automatic external defibrillator is analyzing the rhythm?
    A. The device emits oral messages that might not be heard during CPR.
    B. The device senses the CPR compressions and cannot be turned on.
    C. The device can automatically deliver a series of three rapid shocks.
    D. The device cannot analyze the rhythm while CPR is being performed.

109. The automatic external defibrillator (AED) is considered safer to use than a manual defibrillator because the AED:
    A. produces less electrical energy.
    B. uses adhesive external pads.
    C. cannot shock the rescuers.
    D. can be used safely when wet.

110. While the automated external defibrillator (AED) is performing its rhythm, you should:
    A. continue to ventilate the patient.
    B. auscultate the breath sounds.
    C. check for a carotid pulse.
    D. remain clear of the patient.

111. While transporting a patient becomes pulse-less and apneic. You apply an older model monophasic AED. Before analyzing the rhythm, you must stop the ambulance and:
    A. turn the motor off.
    B. let the throttle idle.
    C. place it in neutral.
    D. shut off all lights.

112. Which of the following would *not* likely interfere with the automated external defibrillator's ability to analyze the patient's cardiac rhythm?
    A. vehicle engine vibration
    B. vehicle interior lighting
    C. movement of the patient
    D. two-way radio transmission

113. You have provided a single defibrillation with the automated external defibrillator and the patient has regained a pulse. Your next immediate action should be to:
    A. assess the blood pressure.
    B. check the patient's breathing status.
    C. perform a focused physical exam.
    D. begin transport of the patient.

114. Most automated external defibrillator (AED) failures are attributed to:
    A. poor personnel training.
    B. improper maintenance.
    C. complicated directions for its use.
    D. adhesive pad failure.

Scenario

Questions 115–117 refer to the following scenario.

You and your partner respond to 812 Elm Street for a person with chest pain. The patient states, "I was drinking beer and mowing the yard when all of a sudden I became sweaty and my chest began to hurt." The patient is a 40-year-old male with a prior history of chest pain; he has no other prior medical history and seems in good health. He describes the pain as "sharp" and points to the midsternal area. He describes the pain as an 8 on the 1-to-10 severity scale. He denies any shortness of breath. His vital signs are blood pressure, 124/88 mmHg; heart rate, 122 breaths/minute; respiration, 20/minute with full chest rise, pulse oximeter reading, 97 percent on room air. His skin is pale, cool, and clammy.

115. Oxygen therapy for this patient should be delivered by:
    A. nasal cannula at 2 lpm.
    B. nonrebreather mask at 15 lpm.
    C. positive pressure ventilations with bag-valve-mask unit.
    D. blow-by oxygen.

116. To help reduce this patient's anxiety, you should reassure him and place him in which position?
    A. the one in which he is most comfortable
    B. a left lateral recumbent (recovery position)
    C. the Trendelenburg (shock position)
    D. a supine position with legs bent at the knees

117. After assessing the patient, you consult medical direction and are instructed to administer nitroglycerin. A few minutes after administering it, your partner advises you that the blood pressure has dropped to 104/76 mmHg and the pulse rate has increased to 128 beats/minute. Your immediate action is to:
    A. remove the tablet quickly because this patient is too sensitive to this drug.
    B. position the patient appropriately because these are early signs of anaphylaxis.

C. reassure the patient, explaining that these are common side effects of nitroglycerin.

D. administer another nitroglycerin to stabilize the condition and increase the blood pressure.

118. In which of the following patients would the use of the automated external defibrillator be indicated?

A. a 60-year-old medical patient who is in respiratory arrest

B. a 7-month-old that is limp, cyanotic and has no breathing

C. a 74-year-old medical patient who has a systolic blood pressure of 84 mmHg

D. a 21-year-old patient with a head injury who is pulseless and breathless

119. Pediatric pads for an automated external defibrillator should be used in patients between the ages of one and:

A. 14.

B. 12.

C. 10.

D. 8.

120. In general, a patient suffering from a cardiac emergency falls into one of two broad categories:

A. unresponsive in cardiac arrest and responsive with chest discomfort.

B. dead on the scene and cardiac arrest.

C. cardiac arrest and unresponsive chest pain.

D. immediate cardiac arrest and delayed cardiac arrest.

121. Patients who complain of chest pain:

A. require the application and use of the automated external defibrillator.

B. require the automated external defibrillator only if they are in respiratory arrest.

C. can deteriorate to cardiac arrest.

D. will go into cardiac arrest within 1 hour.

122. The type of defibrillator that provides complete operation by pushing a single "on" button is a:

A. manual one.

B. semimanual one.

C. fully automated one.

D. semiautomatic one.

123. The delivery of a defibrillation to a patient who is *not* in cardiac arrest can:

A. cause a dangerous disruption of the heart's conduction system.

B. cause the patient to experience a stroke from the muscular contraction.

C. cause a dangerous increase in the patient's blood pressure.

D. improve the oxygen flow to the cornonary arteries.

124. Which of the following is an advantage of the automated external defibrillator over the use of a manual defibrillator?

A. It delivers a less effective shock than the manual defibrillator.

B. It uses less energy than the manual defibrillator.

C. It does not require the EMT's hands to come near the patient during defibrillation.

D. It does not require CPR to be performed between defibrillations.

125. The automated external defibrillator delivers a defibrillation for which "pulseless" cardiac rhythm?

A. asystole

B. ventricular tachycardia

C. agonal

D. pulseless electrical activity

126. You are using an automated external defibrillator to manage a cardiac arrest patient. You are notified that an advanced life support unit is not available. You should begin transport when:
    A. you have delivered a total of four shocks.
    B. the automated external defibrillator has given one "No Shock" message.
    C. the automated external defibrillator has given three "No Shock" messages.
    D. you have delivered a total of two shocks.

127. Which of the following items of the American Heart Association's chain of survival is directly responsible for terminating ventricular fibrillation in the prehospital setting?
    A. immediate recognition and activation
    B. early CPR
    C. rapid defibrillation
    D. effective ALS

128. Frequent practice with the automated external defibrillator is required to:
    A. meet local rules and operating regulations.
    B. meet federal training and recertification requirements.
    C. ensure that the EMT can properly use the device.
    D. meet state training and recertification requirements.

129. Which of the following would be the *least* likely action taken by the medical director who oversees the automated external defibrillator program?
    A. ensuring that the EMS system has all necessary American Heart Association chain of survival links
    B. engaging in a quality assurance/quality improvement program
    C. recommending that only advanced life support units respond to all cardiac arrest calls
    D. reviewing EMTs in a practical skills setting to ensure skill competency

130. In regard to automated external defibrillator (AED) programs, the EMS system's medical director:
    A. should review an audit of all calls in which the AED is used.
    B. does not have to provide any medical oversight because the AED can be used by the public.
    C. must provide online medical direction to EMTs using the AED.
    D. does not need to review any of the AED calls because all of the information is automatically documented.

131. Defibrillation is most successful for patients in cardiac arrest resulting from:
    A. an ischemic stroke.
    B. a hypoglycemic event.
    C. a dysrhythmia associated with coronary artery disease.
    D. an auto accident in which the patient suffered head trauma.

132. A three-year-old child who is in cardiac arrest requires:
    A. immediate application of an adult automated external defibrillator.
    B. automated external defibrillator application only when the rhythm is ventricular tachycardia.
    C. airway and ventilatory management with chest compressions only.
    D. application of an adult automated external defibrillator with pediatric cables and pads.

133. Nitroglycerin is contraindicated if the patient presents with a systolic blood pressure lower than:
   A. 80 mmHg.
   B. 90 mmHg.
   C. 100 mmHg.
   D. 110 mmHg.

134. If there is no relief of pain, nitroglycerin could typically be repeated up to a total of:
   A. two doses.
   B. three doses.
   C. four doses.
   D. five doses.

135. A common side effect associated with the administration of nitroglycerin is:
   A. nausea.
   B. dyspnea.
   C. vomiting.
   D. headache.

136. Which of the following is true regarding automated external defibrillators (AEDs).
   A. It is easier to learn CPR than it is to learn to operate an AED.
   B. AEDs are unable to detect loose leads and false or misleading rhythm readings.
   C. The semi-AED requires no involvement by the operator.
   D. Semiautomated and automated external defibrillators are equally effective.

137. Which signs of cardiac arrest must be present for you to attach an automated external defibrillator to the patient?
   A. no radial pulses and unresponsiveness
   B. unresponsiveness and apnea
   C. unresponsive and no spontaneous eye opening
   D. unresponsive, apnea, and pulselessness

138. You have successfully defibrillated a patient in cardiac arrest. The patient now has a carotid pulse but no spontaneous breathing. Your advanced life support (ALS) backup has been delayed. You should:
   A. remain on-scene and await arrival of the ALS unit.
   B. delay transport until another EMT unit arrives on the scene.
   C. remove the automated external defibrillator, continue to ventilate, and contact medical direction.
   D. continue to treat the patient and transport immediately.

139. You arrive on the scene and find a 65-year-old male patient who has complained of substernal chest pain for the last 10 minutes. The patient has a history of cardiac problems and is prescribed nitroglycerin. He is alert and oriented and states that he took three nitroglycerin tablets with no relief. His vitals signs are blood pressure, 124/90 mmHg; heart rate, 90 beats/minute; and respiration, 18 and full; and skin is pale, cool, and clammy. His pulse oximeter reading is 97 percent while he is on a nonrebreather mask at 15 lpm. You should:
   A. administer up to two additional doses of nitroglycerin.
   B. apply the automated external defibrillator.
   C. conduct a detailed medical exam.
   D. administer 325 mg of aspirin.

140. The patient from question 139 suddenly grabs his chest, closes his eyes, and slumps forward. He is unresponsive to pain and is pulseless and breathless. You attach the automated external defibrillator, and it advises "No Shock." You should immediately:
   A. reassess the breathing.
   B. begin chest compressions.
   C. check the patient's pulse.
   D. reanalyze the rhythm.

141. When the automated external defibrillator advises "Shock," you should:
    A. check the patient's pulse before delivering the shock.
    B. check with medical direction before delivering the shock.
    C. ensure that all personnel are clear of the patient.
    D. ventilate twice before delivering the shock.

Diabetes/Altered Mental Status

142. The apartment manager who called you tells you that he brought the patient his evening meal and found him on the floor unresponsive. Your assessment reveals a male patient who responds to painful stimuli with moaning. His vital signs are blood pressure, 120/68 mmHg; heart rate, 122 beats/minute; 12 respiration/minute with adequate chest rise; and pulse oximeter, 98 percent. His skin is pale, cool, and clammy. Your partner finds a prescription bottle of Micronase on the counter. You should suspect:
    A. a myocardial infarction.
    B. a stroke.
    C. hypoglycemia.
    D. hypothermia.

143. A sign of hypoglycemia is:
    A. a slow onset of altered mental status.
    B. bradycardia.
    C. warm, flushed skin.
    D. pale, cool, clammy skin.

144. To administer instant glucose, a patient must have:
    A. an intact gag reflex and the ability to swallow.
    B. a history of Type I diabetes mellitus.

C. a history of epilepsy controlled by medication.
    D. an altered mental status with a response only to painful stimuli.

145. To properly administer oral glucose, you should:
    A. allow the patient to suck on the tube until the symptoms appear to resolve.
    B. place a pinch between the patient's cheek and gum every 3 to 5 minutes until the symptoms resolve.
    C. place the glucose on a tongue depressor, deposit the glucose between the cheek and gum, and then rub the area.
    D. squirt approximately half of the tube into the patient's mouth and allow it to dissolve.

146. You find a 32-year-old unresponsive female patient. The family states that she is a Type I diabetic. As you approach the patient, you note sonorous sounds. The patient is extremely pale and diaphoretic. You should immediately:
    A. insert an oropharyngeal airway and administer oral glucose.
    B. apply a nonrebreather mask and administer oral glucose.
    C. perform a jaw thrust and assess the radial pulse.
    D. do a head-tilt, chin-lift maneuver and assess the ventilation status.

147. Which of the following is a contraindication to the administration of oral glucose?
    A. the inability to swallow or unconsciousness
    B. a decreased level of consciousness
    C. systolic blood pressure of less than 100 mmHg
    D. headache and diaphoresis

148. Your first priority in managing a patient who has an altered mental status from a diabetic emergency is to:
    A. administer oral glucose.
    B. administer oxygen by nasal cannula.
    C. establish and maintain an open airway.
    D. determine whether the patient can swallow.

149. You are called to the scene for a patient who has an altered mental status. His family states that he has had nothing to eat or drink since around 5:00 P.M. yesterday. It is 7:45 A.M. in the morning. Medical direction asks that you assess the blood glucose level by using a capillary glucose meter. What would you consider a normal blood glucose level in this patient?
    A. 60 to 70 mg/dL
    B. 80 to 90 mg/dL
    C. 100 to 120 mg/dL
    D. 130 to 140 mg/dL

150. Your diabetic patient is unresponsive to verbal stimuli but responds to pain. The respirations are 14/minute with full chest rise. Which of the following emergency care is most appropriate?
    A. Initiate oxygen therapy, place the patient in the Trendelenburg position, and administer oral glucose.
    B. Initiate oxygen therapy, administer oral glucose, and position the patient on his side.
    C. Maintain an open airway, administer oxygen by nasal cannula, and place the patient in a Fowler position.
    D. Maintain an open airway, administer high-flow oxygen, position the patient on his side, and transport him.

151. Which of the following is a correct method to administer oral glucose to a patient with a history of diabetes controlled by medication?
    A. Lift the tongue and squeeze a small amount under the tongue (sublingually).
    B. Hold back the cheek and squeeze the oral glucose between the cheek and gum.
    C. Tip the patient's head backward and squeeze a small amount into the mouth and ask the patient to swallow it.
    D. Place a small amount on the tongue and ask the patient to swallow it at once.

152. While you are administering oral glucose to an insulin-dependent diabetic patient, he becomes unresponsive. You should immediately:
    A. reassess his airway, breathing, and circulation status.
    B. place the patient in a Fowler's position to protect the airway.
    C. try to remove the oral glucose by gently scraping the contents from the cheek.
    D. administer an additional dose to quickly raise the blood glucose level and reverse the unresponsiveness.

153. The priority in managing a patient with an altered mental status is to:
    A. administer oral glucose.
    B. maintain a patent airway.
    C. obtain a blood glucose reading.
    D. complete an early detailed physical exam.

154. Place the following treatment steps in the most appropriate order for an unresponsive patient with diabetes:
    1. Administer oxygen.
    2. Suction secretions.
    3. Obtain a SAMPLE history.
    4. Perform a rapid head-to-toe physical assessment.
    A. 1, 2, 4, 3
    B. 4, 2, 1, 3
    C. 2, 4, 1, 3
    D. 2, 1, 4, 3

155. In what position should you place a patient who has an altered mental status that requires ventilation?
    A. supine
    B. Trendelenburg
    C. lateral recumbent
    D. prone

156. For which patient would oral glucose administration be inappropriate?
    A. Type I insulin-dependent diabetic
    B. Type II noninsulin-dependent diabetic
    C. one with altered mental status who took his insulin 1 hour prior to the onset of the signs and symptoms
    D. one who is in an altered mental status with an intact gag and swallow reflex and is suspected of suffering a stroke

Stroke

157. Which of the following is a common sign of an ischemic stroke?
    A. severe headache
    B. excessive vomiting
    C. difficulty breathing
    D. facial droop

158. The difference between a stroke and transient ischemic attack (TIA) is that:
    A. a TIA usually involves only one side of the body, but a stroke affects both sides.
    B. a stroke usually causes TIAs to occur for long periods of time after the stroke has resolved itself.
    C. the signs and symptoms of a TIA disappear within 24 hours and usually result in no permanent neurologic dysfunction, but a stroke commonly produces permanent signs.
    D. a stroke require transport to a medical facility but a transient ischemic attack does not.

159. You arrive on the scene and find that the patient is unable to move his right arm and has decreased sensation in his right leg. The patient's vital signs are: blood pressure, 193/110 mmHg; heart rate, 112 beats/minute and irregular; respiration, 22 with good chest rise; and pulse oximeter, 93 percent on room air. Your initial treatment should include:
    A. applying a nasal cannula at 2 lpm.
    B. splinting the paralyzed extremities.
    C. ventilating with a bag-valve-mask device.
    D. providing rapid transport to the nearest medical facility.

160. You arrive on the scene and find an unresponsive patient supine on the floor. His wife tells you that he just got back from running and complained of "the worst headache of my life" and then suddenly fell to the ground. You should suspect:
    A. a massive myocardial infarction.
    B. a hemorrhagic stroke.
    C. an ischemic stroke.
    D. a transient ischemic attack.

161. A cerebral embolism most likely originates in:
    A. clotted blood from the inferior vena cava.
    B. stagnant blood from the left side of the heart.
    C. tumor fragments from the right ventricle.
    D. thrombophlebitis from deep vein thrombosis.

162. Which of the following could be a late sign or symptom of a stroke?
    A. slurred speech
    B. headache
    C. paralysis
    D. stiff neck

163. Which of the following would be an unusual sign for a stroke patient?
    A. loss of bowel and bladder control
    B. paralysis to one side of the body
    C. severe intermittent abdominal pain
    D. loss of vision in one or both eyes

164. When managing an ischemic stroke patient, which of the following is critical to report to the receiving medical facility?
    A. the Glasgow Coma Score
    B. the exact time of onset of the first sign or symptom of the stroke
    C. the name of each medication that the patient is taking
    D. all of the findings of the detailed physical exam

Allergic Reactions and Anaphylaxis

165. Which of the following would be unlikely to occur in an allergic reaction?
    A. warm, tingling feeling in the face, mouth, feet, and tongue
    B. decreased heart rate
    C. tightness in the throat and/or the chest
    D. urticaria and pruritis

166. Which would *not* occur during an anaphylactic reaction?
    A. swelling at the level of the larynx, causing airway compromise
    B. constriction and swelling of the inner lining of the bronchioles
    C. dilation of vessels and leakage of capillaries
    D. constriction of vessels in the skin and underlying tissue

167. Your patient was stung by a yellow jacket and now is complaining of difficulty swallowing, shortness of breath, and tightness in the chest. Your primary concern in this patient is to:
    A. provide aggressive airway management with positive pressure ventilation if necessary.
    B. place him in a left lateral recumbent position.
    C. activate advanced life support because of the patient's rapid respiratory deterioration.
    D. apply the automated external defibrillator for impending cardiac arrest.

168. Your patient states that she is "deathly" allergic to peanuts and just ate a pie cooked with peanut oil. She appears to be itching all over and has watery eyes and hives on her chest and arms. The patient has no other complaints. You would classify this as a:
    A. severe reaction and immediately administer epinephrine.
    B. mild reaction and provide positive pressure ventilation and endotracheal intubation.
    C. mild reaction and provide supplemental oxygen and monitor the patient closely.
    D. severe reaction and provide supplemental oxygen and reassurance.

169. It is important to consider all cases of allergic reactions as serious because:
    A. a mild reaction can rapidly progress to severe anaphylaxis.
    B. infection from the stinger of a bee can cause the loss of an extremity.
    C. allergic reactions can mimic other more serious medical emergencies.
    D. the patient could develop urticaria and pruritis.

170. A sign of anaphylactic shock that would cause you to consider epinephrine administration is:
    A. hypotension.
    B. tachycardia.
    C. hives.
    D. flushed skin.

171. Which of the following is a sign of anaphylaxis?
    A. increased systolic blood pressure
    B. bilateral wheezing in all lung fields
    C. pale, cool, clammy skin
    D. extremely dry conjunctiva and nasal mucosa

172. You are assessing a patient who complains of difficult breathing, hives, and itching. During your assessment, you note high-pitched sounds when the patient inhales. You should suspect:
    A. bronchiole constriction and inflammation.
    B. obstruction of the mainstem bronchi.
    C. swelling of the larynx.
    D. fluid in the alveoli.

173. The sign or symptom that typically appears first in an anaphylactic reaction is:
    A. inspiratory crackles or rales.
    B. hives and itching.
    C. hypotension and tachycardia.
    D. stridorous respirations.

174. Epinephrine used by EMTs to manage a patient in anaphylaxis:
    A. is carried on all EMS units.
    B. is a sublingual injection.
    C. does not require an order to administer it.
    D. is prescribed to the patient.

175. You arrive on the scene and find a patient who states that he is allergic to shellfish. He has hives, is itching, and has slightly flushed skin. His blood pressure is 128/78 mmHg, heart rate is 102 beats/minute, and respiration rate is 18 with adequate chest rise. You should do which of these?
    A. administer 0.3 mg of epinephrine by autoinjector
    B. administer high-flow oxygen by nonrebreather mask at 15 lpm
    C. position the patient in a left lateral recumbent position
    D. administer 325 mg of aspirin by having the patient chew the tablet

176. You suspect that your patient is suffering from an anaphylactic reaction and his airway is compromised by a swollen larynx. The most effective method to manage this obstruction is to:
    A. provide positive pressure ventilation.
    B. position the patient's head.
    C. insert an oropharyngeal airway.
    D. suction the upper airway often.

177. Which of the following is the correct administration procedure for a prescribed epinephrine autoinjector?
    A. Push the autoinjector firmly against the patient's upper hip between the thigh and the lower back; hold in place for 1 second.
    B. Push the autoinjector firmly against the patient's upper arm between the elbow and the shoulder; hold in place until half of the vial has been delivered.
    C. Push the autoinjector firmly against the patient's thigh midway between the waist and the knee; hold in place until all of the medication has been delivered.
    D. Push the autoinjector firmly against the patient's lower leg midway between the knee and the ankle; hold in place until all of the medication has been delivered.

178. You have administered epinephrine to an anaphylactic patient who now complains of a headache, dizziness, chest pain, and increased heart rate. You should recognize these signs as:
    A. the incorrect administration of the epinephrine.
    B. an overdose of epinephrine.
    C. the side effects of epinephrine.
    D. an allergic reaction to the epinephrine.

179. Which of the following is a contraindication of epinephrine administration by autoinjection in anaphylaxis?
    A. no contraindications
    B. patient over the age of 60 years
    C. Infants and children under 8 years of age
    D. patient presenting with stridorous respiration

Poisoning/Overdose Emergencies

180. Which of the following signs or symptoms is *least* likely to indicate an overdose?
    A. pale and cool skin
    B. unequal pupils
    C. slow heart rate
    D. abdominal pain

181. Your first priority in providing emergency medical care to a patient who has overdosed on an unknown medication is to:
    A. administer activated charcoal.
    B. identify the medication taken.
    C. administer high-flow oxygen.
    D. establish and maintain a patent airway.

182. While you are transporting a patient who has overdosed on sleeping pills, the respiratory rate decreases from 12 to 8/minute. Your immediate action should be to:
    A. administer activated charcoal.
    B. begin bag-valve-mask ventilation.
    C. administer oxygen by nonrebreather mask.
    D. place the patient in a lateral recumbent position.

183. In which of the following poisoned patients is activated charcoal indicated?
    A. 8-year-old who mistakenly drank liquid bleach less than 1 hour ago
    B. 38-year-old who inhaled carbon monoxide 3 hours ago
    C. 60-year-old who overdosed on blood pressure pills 2 hours ago
    D. 3-year-old who ingested liquid ammonia less than 10 minutes ago

184. The purpose of activated charcoal is to:
    A. increase urinary output, which forcefully eliminates the poison.
    B. speed absorption into the body where it is eliminated quickly.
    C. adsorb the contaminant, inhibiting absorption into the body.
    D. actively neutralize most poisons, rendering them harmless.

185. Which two routes would be the fastest way in which a poison can enter the body?
    A. ingestion and inhalation
    B. inhalation and absorption
    C. injection and ingestion
    D. injection and inhalation

186. By what route does nitroglycerin spray enter the body?
    A. inhalation
    B. ingestion
    C. absorption
    D. injection

187. A patient is suffering an anaphylactic reaction from a yellow jacket bite. By what route did the venom enter the patient's body?
    A. absorption
    B. injection
    C. inhalation
    D. ingestion

188. A patient has a dry powder poison covering both upper extremities and chest. You should:
    A. cover the patient's arms with a burn sheet to preserve the powder for the emergency room.
    B. immediately wash the powder off to prevent further exposure.
    C. brush the powder off and irrigate the contaminated area with large amounts of water.
    D. flush the area with large amounts of water and then brush the remaining poison off.

189. As you pull up to the scene of a possible chlorine leak, you see two victims lying on the ground by a tool shed. Your immediate action should be to:
    A. remove them from the scene to prevent further contamination.
    B. provide high concentration oxygen to them to prevent further hypoxia.
    C. remove only the victim who appears to be in the more serious condition.
    D. retreat to a safe environment uphill and upwind and contact the fire department.

190. You are managing an unresponsive 22-year-old male who overdosed on Valium. To protect the patient's airway, you should:
    A. insert an oropharyngeal airway.
    B. place the patient in a lateral recumbent position.
    C. begin bag-valve-mask ventilation.
    D. decompress the stomach to induce vomiting.

191. In cases of poisoning, your best resource for information regarding treatment of the patient is the:
    A. patient's family physician.
    B. drug/chemical information booklet.
    C. local poison control center.
    D. handheld drug reference.

192. Any poisoning/overdose patient should be transported to a medical facility because:
    A. the effects of the poison could take minutes to hours to days to have severe effects.
    B. you are not capable of protecting the patient's airway in the prehospital setting.
    C. you are concerned that that patient could have a communicable disease that you need to have confirmed.
    D. the patient could become violent and it is better to restrain him in the emergency department than in the ambulance.

193. Your patient has swallowed industrial drain cleaner in a possible suicide attempt. She responds only to deep painful stimuli. Her vital signs are blood pressure, 102/76 mmHg; heart rate, 124 beats/minute; respiration, 42 and shallow; and SpO_2 82 percent. You should:
    A. insert an oropharyngeal airway.
    B. flush the mouth to remove any drain cleaner to prevent further contamination.
    C. apply a nonrebreather mask at 15 lpm.
    D. begin bag-valve-mask ventilation.

194. Which of the following is *not* always part of the assessment or treatment of patient who has overdosed?
    A. Ensure that the airway is patent.
    B. Administer activated charcoal.
    C. Perform a medical assessment.
    D. Administer oxygen.

195. Which of the following is not a trade name for activated charcoal?
    A. CharMed.
    B. InstaChar.

C. Actidose.
D. Liqui-Char.

196. Activated charcoal is indicated for poisoning that occurs only by:
    A. ingestion.
    B. injection.
    C. absorption.
    D. inhalation.

197. For which substance is activated charcoal contraindicated?
    A. digoxin
    B. cental nervous system depressant
    C. oral hypoglycemic
    D. chlorine bleach

198. The medication form of activated charcoal is:
    A. a fine powder for inhalation.
    B. a powder premixed in water to form a slurry.
    C. a solid that is ingested.
    D. a spray that is absorbed under the tongue.

199. The standard dose for activated charcoal is:
    A. 1 gram per kilogram of body weight.
    B. 5 milligrams per kilogram of body weight.
    C. 1 milligram per kilogram of body weight.
    D. 5 grams per kilogram of body weight.

200. When administering activated charcoal, the EMT should:
    A. avoid shaking the contents.
    B. notify medical direction if the patient vomits.
    C. administer it before receiving an online order from medical direction.
    D. have the patient drink it from a covered opaque container.

201. The purpose of activated charcoal is to:
    A. bind to poisons while they are still in the stomach.
    B. flush the poison from the circulatory system.
    C. move the poison quickly through the intestines.
    D. increase the absorption of the poison in the small intestine.

202. The most common side effect following the administration of activated charcoal is:
    A. an increase in the blood pressure.
    B. a decrease in the heart rate.
    C. dark or black stool.
    D. gastrointestinal bleeding.

203. Why is it necessary to contact medical direction early in the management of a patient who has overdosed or ingested poison?
    A. to provide quality assurance information
    B. to control medical liability costs
    C. to follow most state laws
    D. to obtain the most current treatment orders

204. Which of the following would *least* likely indicate that an emergency is due to drugs or alcohol?
    A. empty liquor bottles at the scene
    B. hospital discharge orders with a pain prescription
    C. an unresponsive patient with unequal pupils
    D. open sores and scars to the upper arms

205. Do not use the "Talk-Down Technique" to manage a violent drug patient who has taken:
    A. phencyclidine.
    B. cocaine.
    C. crack.
    D. heroin.

Environmental Emergencies

206. In what way is the majority of heat lost from the body?
    A. convection
    B. conduction
    C. evaporation
    D. radiation

207. Taking into consideration the process of conduction and water chill, how much faster will cold water cool the body than air?
    A. 100 times
    B. 200 times
    C. 240 times
    D. 275 times

208. Which of the following is a late sign of hypothermia?
    A. muscle stiffness
    B. slow heart rate
    C. uncoordination
    D. pale skin

209. When a patient is immersed in water that has the same temperature as that of the ambient air, the body core temperature will:
    A. drop 25 to 30 times faster in the water than in the ambient air.
    B. stay the same as the temperature of the ambient air regardless of the temperature of the water.
    C. drop 100 times faster in the water than in the ambient air.
    D. not drop as fast as it does in the ambient air because the water acts as to insulate body heat.

210. Why are patients who are elderly more pre-disposed to heat emergencies?
    A. They suffer from early stages of congestive heart failure.
    B. They often have kidney failure and are on dialysis.
    C. They typically have a poor fluid intake and are commonly dehydrated.
    D. They typically take an aspirin each day that thins the blood.

211. The priority in managing the patient suffering from a heat emergency who has hot dry skin is to:
    A. remove the patient from the hot environment.
    B. place the patient in an ice bath.
    C. place the patient in a Trendelenburg position.
    D. cover the patient with blankets to prevent cooling too rapidly.

212. A likely cause of continued respiratory distress in a patient who was submerged in the ocean for 5 minutes prior to being resuscitated is:
    A. a myocardial infarction.
    B. congestive heart failure.
    C. head injury from a shallow water dive.
    D. aspiration of salt water.

213. Bystanders pulled a young man from the water who is now sitting on the beach coughing up small amounts of water. He states that he does not believe he needs to go to the hospital because he swallowed only a small amount of water. What should you do?
    A. Agree with the patient because a small amount of water is not harmful.
    B. Explain to the patient that if he wants to, he can go to the hospital in his friend's car.
    C. Explain to the patient the implications involved with a near drowning and attempt to convince him to allow you to transport him to the emergency department to be evaluated.
    D. Have him make an appointment to see his family physician the next day after the incident.

214. Infants and young children lose heat more quickly than adults because they:
    A. are smaller in size but have a larger surface area.
    B. have hyperactive thermoregulatory controls.
    C. have a higher fat content than that of an adult.
    D. have a metabolism much slower than that of an adult.

215. Which of the following is appropriate emergency care for the patient with severe generalized hypothermia?
    A. Transfer, move, or handle the patient as you would any other patient.
    B. Provide only one defibrillation if the patient is in cardiac arrest.
    C. Rub or massage the patient's arms or legs to increase the heat production.
    D. Hyperventilate the patient at a rate of 24/minute to maximize oxygenation.

216. If you cannot detect a pulse or respiration in a patient with severe hypothermia but he moves, you should:
    A. start CPR immediately.
    B. start CPR and apply the automated external defibrillator immediately.
    C. begin positive pressure ventilation.
    D. apply the automated external defibrillator to determine the patient's rhythm.

217. When actively rewarming a patient with hypothermia, the patient's temperature should not be increased by more than how many degree(s) Fahrenheit per hour?
    A. 0.5
    B. 1
    C. 2
    D. 3

218. Which of the following is appropriate management for a patient with immersion hypothermia?
    A. Instruct the patient to swim and tread water as vigorously as possible.
    B. Lift the patient from the water in a horizontal position.
    C. Place the patient in a Trendelenburg position immediately upon removing him from the water.
    D. Leave the wet clothing on the patient to insulate him from heat loss upon removal from the water.

219. Which emergency care should be provided to a patient with a localized cold injury?
    A. Massage the cold tissue.
    B. Remove jewelry to prevent a tourniquet effect.
    C. Apply a salve or ointment to open wounds.
    D. Break blisters that are present on the surface of the skin.

220. Rewarming localized frozen tissue:
    A. is safe to perform on all patients.
    B. can be safely performed by using dry heat.
    C. requires water of 120 to 130 degrees Fahrenheit.
    D. is extremely painful for the patient.

221. You are treating a patient who was stung by a wasp. Which of the following would be an appropriate step in the emergency care?
    A. Remove the stinger using tweezers or your fingers.
    B. Elevate the injection site above the level of the heart.
    C. Wash the area around the sting site with soap.
    D. Apply a hot pack to the injection site to relieve swelling.

Scenario

Questions 222–224 refer to the following scenario:

You are called to an excavation site for a man down on a hot summer day. You find a 40-year-old unresponsive male patient. A worker at the site stated that the patient began to act unusual and then "passed out." His vital signs are blood pressure, 92/70 mmHg; heart rate, 112 beats/minute, regular and strong; and respiration, 24/minute, deep and rapid. His skin is hot and dry.

222. You should immediately:
    A. begin bag-valve-mask ventilation.
    B. apply cold packs to the neck, axillary region, and groin.
    C. place the patient in a lateral recumbent position.
    D. move the patient to a cooler environment.

223. What condition does the patient most likely have?
    A. heat stroke
    B. stroke
    C. heat exhaustion
    D. hyperglycemia

224. The skin signs most likely indicate that:
    A. the patient is experiencing a mild form of a heat emergency.
    B. the relative humidity of the ambient air must be low.
    C. severe hypoxia is in an early stage.
    D. the patient became dehydrated from excessive sweating.

225. Which of the following increases the patient's risk of becoming hypothermic?
    A. alcohol intoxication
    B. a family member who once became hypothermic
    C. a high sensitivity to cold
    D. middle age

226. A compensatory mechanism found early in a hypothermic patient to maintain body temperature is:
    A. bradycardia.
    B. increased respiratory rate.
    C. shivering.
    D. decreased fine motor function.

227. You are treating a 54-year-old female patient who was working in the garden in the hot sun for several hours. She is alert and responding appropriately. She complains of weakness, muscle cramps, and lightheadedness. Her vital signs are blood pressure, 96/70 mmHg; heart rate, 124 beats/minute; and respiration, 16/minute with good chest rise. Her skin is moist, pale, and cool. You should:
    A. have the patient drink cool water.
    B. place the patient in a lateral recumbent position.
    C. apply ice packs to the neck, groin, and axillary regions.
    D. administer one tube of oral glucose.

228. When managing a patient who was bitten by a rattlesnake, you should:
    A. apply cold packs to the injection site.
    B. lower the injection site below the level of the heart.
    C. attempt to suck out the venom from the bite.
    D. Apply a tourniquet to stop circulation to the extremity.

229. You should remove a stinger by:
    A. squeezing it with a pair of tweezers.
    B. scraping it free with the edge of a knife or credit card.
    C. pulling it free with your fingers.
    D. making a small incision through the site and suctioning it free.

Scenario

Questions 230–232 refer to the following scenario:

You and your partner Ashley are restocking the ambulance after a serious automobile accident on I-95. The station alerting system sounds, "Unit one respond to an allergic reaction at 1729 17th Avenue. Time out 13:52." As you approach the scene, you are met at the street by a frantic man who states, "It's my wife; she was stung by a bee and now she can't breathe." You and Ashley enter the house and find a 36-year-old female sitting on a kitchen chair. She is in a tripod position and looks at you and Ashley with frightened eyes. She is breathing approximately 40 times a minute with shallow chest rise. Ashley states that she can hear audible wheezes; the patient's skin is flushed and dry with urticaria (hives) covering the face, neck, chest, and back. The patient begins to slump over the chair. Her heart rate is 134 beats/minute. The SpO_2 is 84 percent on room air. Her blood pressure is 88/62 mmHg.

230. You should immediately:
   A. place a constricting band above the injection site.
   B. wash the injection site.
   C. begin bag-valve-mask ventilation.
   D. apply a nonrebreather mask at 15 lpm.

231. The patient's husband locates and gives you her epinephrine autoinjector. You should next:
   A. administer the patient's prescribed epinephrine by autoinjector.
   B. withhold the epinephrine autoinjector until the blood pressure falls to 80 mmHg systolic.
   C. administer 325 mg of aspirin and wait for a relief in the wheezing.
   D. wait until the heart rate decreases to less than 120 beats/minute prior to administering the epinephrine.

232. After you have administered epinephrine by autoinjector, the patient becomes pale and very anxious and states that she feels as if she is going to vomit. Her heart rate increases to 150 beats/minute. You should suspect that:
   A. you have administered too much epinephrine.
   B. these are common side effects of epinephrine.
   C. a second anaphylactic reaction is occurring.
   D. you have administered a bad batch of epinephrine.

Psychiatric Emergencies

233. The way a person acts, including any and all physical and mental activity, is a definition of:
   A. anxiety.
   B. behavior.
   C. depression.
   D. morals and ethics.

234. A behavioral emergency is best defined as:
   A. behavior that is unethical.
   B. behavior that does not represent what the prudent person would do in certain situations.
   C. behavior that is "abnormal" in the given situation and intolerable to the patient, community, or family.
   D. any situation that requires a psychiatric consultation.

235. What condition could produce signs and symptoms similar to that of a behavioral emergency?
   A. hypovolemia
   B. anaphylaxis
   C. collapsed lung
   D. head injury

236. You are called to the scene for a patient who was struck by an automobile. There are no witnesses, and the driver states that the patient came out of nowhere. En route to the hospital, the patient states that all he wanted to do was to die. Your reaction to this comment should be to:
   A. assume that the patient has suffered severe head trauma and is incoherent.
   B. assume that the patient is intoxicated and does not know what he is saying.
   C. pay no attention to the remark because the patient could be delirious from the accident or suffering a head injury.
   D. report the statement to the nurse and physician because the accident could have been a suicide attempt.

237. Risk factors that suggest suicidal tendencies include:
   A. recent marriage.
   B. ages of 17 through 30.
   C. loss of a significant loved one.
   D. recent promotion with additional stress.

238. Approximately what percentage of patients who have succeeded in committing suicide made previous attempts?
    A. 90 percent
    B. 80 percent
    C. 50 percent
    D. 40 percent

239. During the assessment of a despondent patient, you notice multiple cuts on the victim's wrists and arms. You should be concerned that the patient:
    A. could have been involved in a fight.
    B. could have been tied up for a period of time.
    C. could have attempted suicide.
    D. is an IV drug user and possibly HIV positive.

240. When you are assessing suicidal tendencies, what is the likelihood that the patient with a realistic and concrete plan will commit suicide as compared to the person who has no plan or one that is vague?
    A. less likely
    B. more likely
    C. equally likely
    D. none for either

241. When a patient tells you that he has thought of harming himself with a gun, you should:
    A. do nothing because this is just a way to gain attention.
    B. make sure that the patient is not armed and is not a danger to you.
    C. ask the patient to show you the gun because this will prove his intentions.
    D. attempt to console the patient and find out why he wants to hurt himself.

242. You are called to a private residence for an unknown emergency. You walk into the residence and find an elderly man sitting among bottles of whiskey and crying over a

picture. You observe a pistol in the patient's waistband. Your first action should be to:
    A. ask the patient why he is so sad.
    B. determine whether the patient wants to kill himself.
    C. slowly and calmly back out of the room.
    D. charge the patient and restrain him.

243. Which is an inaccurate description of a high risk for suicide?
    A. A patient who has a substance abuse problem is more likely to commit suicide.
    B. Older individuals usually are more mature and less likely to commit suicide.
    C. Females are less likely to commit suicide than are males.
    D. A patient who describes a definite plan for the suicide is more likely to commit it.

244. In which situation is the EMT most likely to be injured from violence?
    A. when arriving on the scene of a stabbing or shooting
    B. when the patient has threatened to commit suicide
    C. when the patient is homeless and hungry
    D. when the patient's behavior changes rapidly

245. If you suspect that your patient is a suicide risk and does not want to go to the hospital, what should you *not* do while at the scene?
    A. Call medical direction and ask for permission to restrain the patient.
    B. Allow the patient to go to the bedroom alone to collect his clothes.
    C. Contact dispatch for additional assistance if restraint is necessary.
    D. Request the police if medical direction orders you to restrain and transport.

246. Which of the following is a risk factor for suicide?
    A. male patient in his mid-20s
    B. arrest or imprisonment even for minor offenses
    C. recent marriage
    D. promotion in current job

247. Which condition is likely to cause the patient to become aggressive?
    A. fear
    B. anxiety
    C. hypoglycemia
    D. all of the above

248. Which of the following is most appropriate when assessing and managing a patient with suicidal intentions?
    A. Explain to the patient that his feelings are not normal and he should not feel that way.
    B. Ask the patient if he wants to commit suicide and how he would do it.
    C. Lie to the patient if necessary to get the patient to cooperate.
    D. To be cautious and protect yourself, restrain the patient regardless of his intent to harm you.

249. You have restrained a patient who was exhibiting violent behavior toward his family. While en route to the hospital, the patient calms down and wants the restraints removed. You should:
    A. remove the restraints if the patient states he is no longer violent.
    B. not remove the restraints for your own safety.
    C. remove the leg restraints only and see how the patient responds.
    D. remove the wrist restraints only for a short time and monitor the patient's behavior.

Acute Abdominal Pain

250. The patient complaining of abdominal pain would concern you the most is the one who:
    A. walks out to the ambulance informing you he has the worst "belly ache."
    B. is sitting upright in a chair, moaning in pain, and drinking antacid.
    C. is rolling about on the floor complaining of pain.
    D. is lying on the floor very still and quiet with his knees drawn up to his chest.

251. Organs of the right upper quadrant include:
    A. pancreas, spleen, and part of the liver.
    B. most of the liver, gallbladder, and part of the large intestine.
    C. small intestine, stomach, and spleen.
    D. most of the liver, spleen, and gallbladder.

252. Your patient was diagnosed with cholecystitis (gallbladder inflammation) three days ago. The patient now presents with nausea, vomiting, and pain in the right shoulder. The pain in the shoulder can be classified as:
    A. referred pain.
    B. visceral pain.
    C. pancreatic pain.
    D. somatic pain.

253. You arrive on the scene to find an approximately 60-year-old male patient writhing on the floor. He is complaining of a tearing pain radiating to his lower back. He has absent femoral pulses and has a pulsatile mass just superior to his umbilicus. You suspect which of the following conditons?
    A. myocardial infarction
    B. abdominal aortic aneurysm
    C. acute pancreatitis
    D. ruptured appendix

254. You are called to a residential neighborhood at 12:30 A.M. Your patient has just finished eating a super-size meal of deep fried fish. He now is complaining of a "crampy" pain in the right upper quadrant and has had two episodes of nausea and vomiting with a green emesis. What condition do you suspect that your patient is experiencing?
    A. a peptic ulcer
    B. an intestinal obstruction
    C. cholecystitis
    D. appendicitis

255. Pain that the patient feels in a body part or area of the body that has nothing to do with a diseased organ is termed:
    A. epigastric pain.
    B. abdominal pain.
    C. retroperitenal pain.
    D. referred pain.

256. Which condition is most likely to cause abdominal pain?
    A. pneumonia
    B. intestinal obstruction
    C. hypoglycemia
    D. stroke

257. A 46-year-old male patient presents with a complaint of severe acute abdominal pain and signs of hypoperfusion. In which position should you place the patient?
    A. lateral recumbent
    B. sitting upright
    C. supine with feet elevated
    D. one of comfort

258. In what position should the patient complaining of severe abdominal pain be placed if there are no signs or symptoms of shock?
    A. supine with feet elevated
    B. one of comfort
    C. left lateral recumbent
    D. semi-Fowler with knees bent

259. When treating a patient with acute abdominal pain, you should do which of these?
    A. have him take antacids in an attempt to decrease the pain
    B. administer sips of water if patient complains of thirst
    C. have the him drink milk to coat the stomach and reduce the pain
    D. have the patient lie still and assume a position of comfort

Obstetrics and Gynecology

260. Which organ houses the developing fetus until birth?
    A. cervix
    B. placenta
    C. uterus
    D. fallopian tubes

261. What organ in pregnancy is responsible for transport of oxygen and nutrients to the fetus and the elimination of carbon dioxide and other waste products?
    A. amniotic sac
    B. placenta
    C. cervix
    D. fallopian tubes

262. You arrive at the scene and find your patient lying on the bed, moaning in pain. She tells you that she is nine months pregnant and is having contractions 2 minutes apart that last for 45 seconds and has the urge to move her bowels. As your partner prepares the obstetrical kit, your next immediate action should be to:
    A. prepare for immediate transport because her labor could last for hours.
    B. assess for crowning.
    C. perform a detailed physical exam.
    D. have the patient put her legs together to delay the delivery until she reaches the hospital.

263. Approximately how far from the infant's abdomen should the first clamp be placed on the umbilical cord?
   A. 12 inches
   B. 10 inches
   C. 6 inches
   D. 2 inches

264. What body substance isolation precautions should be taken when you are preparing to perform a field delivery?
   A. gloves, eye protection, and head nets
   B. mask, gloves, and foot protectors
   C. gown, gloves, and mask
   D. mask, gown, gloves, and eye protection

265. Approximately how far from the first clamp should the second clamp be placed on the umbilical cord?
   A. 1 inch
   B. 3 inches
   C. 6 inches
   D. 10 inches

266. After drying the neonate, his respirations remained depressed. You should immediately:
   A. begin chest compressions.
   B. administer blow-by oxygen.
   C. begin bag-valve-mask ventilation.
   D. stimulate the neonate by flicking the soles of the feet.

267. When should chest compressions be started in the neonate?
   A. when the systolic blood pressure drops below 90 mmHg
   B. when the respirations are weak and not effective
   C. when the heart rate decreases below 60 beats/minute
   D. when the color of the core of the body is cyanotic

268. A foul smelling, greenish brown thick viscous fluid that could be present in the amniotic fluid is:
   A. afterbirth.
   B. meconium.
   C. dried blood.
   D. the bloody show.

269. Meconium is an indication of:
   A. precipitative delivery.
   B. poor prenatal care.
   C. fetal distress.
   D. congenital deformities.

270. When meconium is present in the amniotic fluid or in the neonate's airway, you should:
   A. stimulate the neonate immediately to allow full expansion of his lungs to prevent fetal hypoxia.
   B. immediately warm and stimulate the neonate because the meconium can depress his ability to warm himself.
   C. help stimulate the neonate's cough reflex to allow removal of the meconium from the lungs.
   D. immediately suction the airway before providing any other treatment including stimulation.

271. The perineum is the:
   A. area between the vagina and the anus.
   B. organ to which the umbilical cord is attached.
   C. opening of the uterus.
   D. lateral aspects of the vagina.

272. You are delivering a baby and notice a thick viscous fluid all over the baby and a foul smell. Your immediate reaction and treatment should be to:

A. finish the delivery and activate advanced life support immediately.

B. begin to suction the baby's mouth and nose immediately.

C. wait for the placenta to deliver before you begin cleaning the baby off.

D. do nothing because this is a normal event.

273. You just delivered a neonate who required bag-valve-mask ventilation due to a depressed respiratory status. Upon reassessment, you determine that the infant's heart rate is 138/minute, respirations are 38/minute with adequate chest rise, and the skin is pink. You should:

A. apply deep orotracheal suction to remove any possible secretions and continue ventilation.

B. gradually decrease the rate and volume of each ventilation over 1 minute.

C. hyperventilate the neonate for 1 full minute before stopping ventilation.

D. stop ventilation and reassess the neonate in 1 to 2 minutes.

274. What is the compression to ventilation ratio for neonatal CPR?

A. 120 compressions to 30 ventilations per minute

B. 30 compressions to 90 ventilations per minute

C. 100 compressions to 30 ventilations per minute

D. 90 compressions to 30 ventilations per minute

275. The correct depth for chest compressions in a newborn is:

A. one-half the depth of the chest.

B. one-fourth to three-fourths of an inch in depth.

C. one-fourth to one-half of an inch in depth.

D. one-third of the depth of the chest.

276. When ventilating a newborn, you should reassess the response to ventilation every:

A. 30 seconds.

B. 2 minutes.

C. 3 minutes.

D. 5 minutes.

277. You are called to the scene for a 32-year-old patient who is seven months pregnant and complaining of lightheadedness and feeling faint when she lies flat on her back. Upon your arrival, you find the patient lying supine in bed. She is alert but responds sluggishly to your questions. She is slightly pale, cool, and clammy. She is likely suffering from:

A. preeclampsia.

B. eclampsia.

C. abruptio placenta.

D. supine hypotensive syndrome.

278. A 25-year-old female patient presents with steady vaginal bleeding. You should:

A. perform an internal exam of the vagina to determine the cause of bleeding.

B. place a sanitary pad over the vaginal opening to collect the blood.

C. pack the vagina with sterile gauze to control excessive blood loss.

D. place the patient in a Fowler's position.

279. Delivery of the fetal tissue before the 20th week of gestation is termed:

A. placenta previa.

B. abruptio placenta.

C. breech presentation.

D. spontaneous abortion.

280. During your assessment of a mother who is in labor, you should not allow her to:
  A. walk around the room in an attempt to decrease the pain.
  B. lie in a lateral recumbent position.
  C. breathe deeply and quickly with each contraction.
  D. use the bathroom when she has the urge to defecate.

281. Which of the following is not a standard piece of equipment found in the obstetrical kit carried on the ambulance?
  A. bulb syringe
  B. plastic bag with ties
  C. bag-valve-mask
  D. cord clamps or cord ties

282. As soon as the neonate's head is delivered:
  A. quickly provide aggressive uterine massage.
  B. suction the mouth first and then the nose.
  C. begin bag-valve-mask ventilation.
  D. suction the nose first and then the mouth.

283. During delivery of the neonate's head:
  A. the cord should not be removed from around the neck until after the entire body have been delivered.
  B. the amniotic sac should be kept intact.
  C. grasp firmly under the neonate's arms to deliver the shoulders.
  D. avoid excessive pressure over the fontanel area of the head.

284. Following delivery of the neonate's head, you should immediately:
  A. create a sterile field around the vaginal opening.
  B. determine whether the umbilical cord is around his neck.
  C. record the time of delivery on the medical report.
  D. stimulate the fetus by rubbing its head.

285. How much blood loss is considered to be normal during childbirth and typically well tolerated by the mother?
  A. 100 mL
  B. 300 mL
  C. 500 mL
  D. 700 mL

286. Uterine massage is performed to:
  A. increase the uterus size by smooth muscle relaxation.
  B. stimulate milk production.
  C. reduce uterine contractions.
  D. stimulate contraction of the uterine smooth muscle.

287. In a multiple birth (twins, triplets):
  A. each neonate always has its own placenta.
  B. the neonates always share a placenta.
  C. neonates can have their own placenta or share one.
  D. the placenta is abnormally large.

288. In multiple births, about how many of the deliveries of the second infant are breech?
  A. one-half
  B. one-fifth
  C. three-quarters
  D. one-third

289. Place in the correct sequence the following steps for the treatment of the patient with an injury to the external female genitalia.
    1. ensure airway, breathing, and circulation
    2. provide transportation
    3. care for bleeding from the vagina
    4. administer oxygen

    A. 1, 3, 4, 2
    B. 3, 1, 4, 2
    C. 1, 4, 3, 2
    D. 4, 1, 3, 2

290. You have responded to a vehicle accident. Upon arrival, you observe a pregnant patient who is the unrestrained driver of the vehicle. She was involved in a low-speed accident in a parking lot at the grocery store. She tells you that she struck the back end of a car while traveling about 15 miles per hour. She is about a week from her due date. The patient refuses transport. When assessing for evidence of hypoperfusion, you should:
    A. expect the blood pressure to fall quickly.
    B. not bother checking peripheral perfusion.
    C. realize that signs of shock can be subtle and the patient can deteriorate quickly.
    D. rely on the blood pressure as the best evidence of blood loss.

291. If the pregnant patient in question 290 begins complaining of lower abdominal pain, which of the following questions would be *least* important when obtaining a history of the present illness from this patient?
    A. How intense is the pain?
    B. What is the quality of the pain?

C. Is the pain constant?
D. Do you take any over-the-counter medications?

292. The pregnant patient in her third trimester complains of intermittent abdominal pain that occurs about every 2 minutes and lasts for about 1 minute. Her abdomen is very rigid on palpation. She tells you that she needs to use the bathroom. After completing the primary assessment, you should immediately:
    A. allow the patient to use the bathroom.
    B. transport her rapidly because early signs of shock are present.
    C. evaluate her for crowning.
    D. place her in a supine position with the legs elevated.

293. The initial suctioning of a newborn's mouth and nose with a bulb syringe should be performed:
    A. immediately after the cutting the umbilical cord.
    B. as soon as the entire delivery is completed.
    C. as soon as the head is delivered.
    D. directly after the torso is delivered.

294. When initially removing fluids from a newborn's airway during the birth process, you should:
    A. place the bulb syringe into position and then compress the bulb.
    B. suction the mouth first and then the nose.
    C. advance the tip of the bulb syringe until it touches the back of the pharynx.
    D. stimulate the newborn prior to removing fluid with the bulb syringe.

295. To prevent supine hypotensive syndrome in the pregnant patient in her third trimester, you should:

A. place her on her back with her knees bent.

B. place her in a prone position.

C. place her in a supine position with her legs elevated.

D. elevate her right hip with a pillow or blanket roll.

296. You are treating a pregnant patient in her eighth month for a generalized seizure. You should first:

A. transport her immediately using lights and siren.

B. administer high-flow oxygen by nonrebreather mask.

C. position this postictal patient lying on her left side.

D. suction any blood or secretions from the mouth.

297. Which emergency care would be inappropriate and may cause injury when assisting the delivery of a newborn?

A. Tear the amniotic sac with your fingers if it has not ruptured during crowning.

B. If bleeding appears heavy after delivery, massage the mother's abdomen.

C. Place the first umbilical clamp approximately 6 inches from the infant's abdomen.

D. Apply pressure to the fontanel to prevent an explosive delivery.

298. When delivering the placenta, you should:

A. grasp it and guide it once it begins to be expelled from the vagina.

B. apply firm pressure to the umbilical cord to facilitate the placenta delivery.

C. remain on scene until the placenta and attached membranes have been delivered.

D. place the placenta and membranes in a biohazard bag and dispose of it at the hospital.

299. In which emergency setting is it permissible to insert your gloved hand into the pregnant patient's vagina?

A. a prolapsed cord

B. abruptio placenta

C. arm or leg presentation

D. multiple births

300. When you assess a pregnant patient who is in labor for crowning, you note that the fetus's arm is protruding from the vaginal opening. You should:

A. place the mother in a head-down supine position with her pelvis elevated and transport her immediately.

B. cover the limb with a moist sterile dressing and continue with the delivery as normal.

C. place your gloved hand into the vagina and maneuver the fetus into position.

D. gently push the limb back into the vagina while applying pressure back on the fetus.

301. Which characteristic indicates that an infant is premature?

A. The infant has coarse hair.

B. The sole of the foot has many creases.

C. The infant's outer ear has no cartilage.

D. The infant weighs 6.5 pounds at birth.

302. Which emergency care is a priority for a neonate born in the 34th week of pregnancy?
   A. Provide high-flow oxygen by nonrebreather mask to the newborn.
   B. Immediately dry and place the newborn in warmed blankets.
   C. Suction secretions with a tonsil tip catheter.
   D. Obtain a blood glucose level.

Scenario

Questions 303–305 refer to the following scenario:

You and your partner Jim are refueling your vehicle when dispatch alerts you to a woman in active labor. You quickly secure the fuel pump and respond to the emergency. Upon arrival at the scene, you find a 23-year-old female lying supine on her bed. The amniotic sac has ruptured and she feels as if she must push. Jim quickly inspects the vagina for crowning and finds the pulsating umbilical cord protruding.

303. In which position should you and Jim place this patient?
   A. prone with chest elevated with pillows
   B. supine with the hips elevated with pillows
   C. semisitting with knees bent slightly
   D. lying flat on the right side with knees bent

304. While rapidly transporting this patient to the hospital, you notice that the baby's head appears to be pushing against the pulsating umbilical cord. You should immediately:
   A. place a gloved hand into the vagina and gently push the head back and away from the cord.
   B. with your gloved hand, gently pull the cord away from the baby's head.
   C. with your gloved hand, gently push the pulsating cord back into the vagina.
   D. place a gloved hand into the vagina and push the vaginal wall away from the cord.

305. After applying pressure against the fetal head, you observe that the mother is breathing 42 times/minute with shallow breathing. You should immediately:
   A. provide oxygen by nasal cannula at 6 lpm.
   B. provide oxygen by nonrebreather mask at 15 lpm.
   C. open the airway and begin positive pressure ventilation.
   D. place the patient supine and elevate her right hip.

Seizures and Syncope

306. A sudden and temporary alteration in behavior caused by the massive electrical discharge from active foci in a neuron or group of neurons in the brain is a:
   A. stroke.
   B. seizure.
   C. TIA.
   D. cerebral hemorrhage.

307. The pattern or sequence of events for a generalized tonic-clonic seizure includes:
   A. seizure, aura, postictal state.
   B. aura, clonic phase, tonic phase, postictal state.
   C. aura, tonic phase, myotonic phase, postictal state.
   D. aura, tonic phase, clonic phase, postictal state.

308. Which of the following is a likely cause of a seizure?
    A. hyperventilation
    B. panic attack
    C. hyperglycemia
    D. hypoxia

309. Treatment for a patient who is actively seizing includes:
    A. protecting and positioning the patient, maintaining an airway, administering oral glucose, suctioning the airway, and applying supplemental oxygen.
    B. protecting and positioning the patient, prying the mouth open to insert an oral airway, suctioning the airway, applying supplemental oxygen, and providing rapid transport.
    C. protecting and positioning the patient, maintaining an airway, suctioning the airway, assisting ventilations if necessary, applying supplemental oxygen, and transporting.
    D. protecting and positioning the patient, maintaining an airway, suctioning the airway, assisting ventilations if needed, applying supplemental oxygen, waiting for the patient to regain consciousness to sign a refusal form.

310. A patient having seizures lasting more than 5 minutes or seizures that occur without a period of consciousness between is considered to be suffering from:
    A. a grand mal seizure.
    B. tonic-clonic seizures.
    C. status epilepticus.
    D. a prolonged hysterical seizure.

311. The tonic phase of a seizure is identified by:
    A. loss of consciousness.
    B. rigid muscles.
    C. jerky muscle movement.
    D. loss of bowel control.

312. The tonic-clonic phase of a seizure is recognized by:
    A. muscles alternate between rigidity and relaxation, producing a jerky movement.
    B. loss of bowel and bladder control.
    C. shrill and high-pitched sounds made during the muscular movement.
    D. hyperventilation and tachycardia.

313. The preferred airway adjunct for a patient who is actively seizing status epilepticus and whose teeth are clenched is the:
    A. nasopharyngeal airway.
    B. oropharyngeal airway.
    C. endotracheal tube.
    D. combitube.

314. A common medication used in the treatment of epilepsy or a seizure disorder is:
    A. digoxin.
    B. phenytoin sodium.
    C. diphenhydramine.
    D. Versed.

315. A patient who suffers two or more consecutive seizures without a period of consciousness between them or a seizure that lasts longer than 5 minutes has a condition referred to as:
    A. continual epilepsy.
    B. continual seizure.
    C. status epilepticus.
    D. status seizure.

316. Which of the following statements is true regarding syncope?
    A. The episode usually occurs when the patient is supine.
    B. The patient does not remember feeling faint or lightheaded.
    C. The patient becomes responsive quickly after being positioned supine.
    D. The patient remembers an abnormal sound, odor, or visual disturbance.

317. The patient with a history of epilepsy suddenly states that she is experiencing a metallic taste in her mouth, which she says is an aura. She will next likely experience:

A. a postictal state.

B. a petit mal seizure.

C. a generalized tonic-clonic seizure.

D. a focal motor seizure.

318. The convulsion phase that presents with typical violent and jerky muscle movement is known as the:

A. hypertonic phase.

B. tonic-clonic phase.

C. tonic phase.

D. postictal phase.

319. Which phase of a seizure is known as the *recovery phase* during which the patient's mental status progressively improves over time?

A. postictal phase

B. tonic phase

C. clonic phase

D. aura phase

320. A typical syncopal episode (faint) usually begins while the patient is in which position?

A. lying

B. kneeling

C. standing

D. sitting

321. When providing emergency care to a patient who has experienced a syncopal episode, you should place this patient in which position?

A. sitting with head between the knees

B. supine with the legs elevated

C. prone with the head elevated

D. Fowler with the feet elevated

322. A bystander states that the patient was standing when he became pale and diaphoretic and began to yawn and sway. He then became unresponsive and fell to the ground. After the patient fell to the ground, he immediately became responsive again. You suspect that the patient experienced:

A. a generalized seizure.

B. a syncopal episode.

C. a heart attack.

D. a hypoglycemic event.

323. A patient who is postictal following a tonic-clonic seizure is displaying obvious right-sided weakness upon assessment. There is no obvious trauma to the patient. The family states that is a normal seizure for him. You should recognize that:

A. a stroke likely occurred during the seizure.

B. a heart attack is the cause of the seizure.

C. the patient likely struck his head during the seizure and now has a head injury.

D. the weakness or paralysis is transient and can be a normal postictal response.

324. A febrile seizure is considered serious if it lasted longer than:

A. 3 minutes.

B. 5 minutes.

C. 10 minutes.

D. 15 minutes.

325. A patient with a history of epilepsy complains of a sharp pain in his abdomen prior to suffering a tonic-clonic seizure. The abdominal pain would best be described as:

A. abdominal bleeding that caused the seizure.

B. an aura that indicated the seizure was imminent.

C. a postictal symptom associated with the seizure.

D. a result of the medication to control the seizure.

General Pharmacology

1.
B. Activated charcoal, oral glucose, and oxygen are medications that EMT units carry. Activated charcoal is no longer carried on some EMS units because of the change in the management of poisoned patients. An epinephrine autoinjector, nitroglycerin, and beta 2 inhaler are not typically carried on the ambulance but are prescribed to and carried by the patient. The EMT is allowed to assist with these medications.

2.
D. EMTs can assist with the administration of epinephrine by autoinjector for anaphylaxis, a beta 2 specific drug by metered-dose inhaler for respiratory emergencies, and nitroglycerin for cardiac emergencies if the prescription is for the patient, there are no contraindications, and medical direction authorizes the procedure.

3.
A. The EMT is allowed to assist the patient in taking prescribed beta 2 agonist drugs that are designed to relax the bronchiole smooth muscle.

Albuterol is a beta 2 agonist drug. Atrovent is ipatropium bromide, a drug used to relax the bronchiole smooth muscle in patients suffering from respiratory diseases; however, it does this through an anticholinergic effect, not beta 2 stimulation. Because it is not a beta 2 agonist, ipatropium bromide is not one of the drugs with which the EMT can assist the patient in taking.

4.
B. Actidose and SuperChar are trade names for activated charcoal, which is used to bind with certain toxic substances in the stomach to limit the amount of poison being absorbed by the gastrointestinal tract. The use of activated charcoal in a patient who has been poisoned has been shown not to be as effective as once thought to be. Many EMS systems have removed activated charcoal from the drugs used by the EMT. Follow your local protocol.

5.
C. The generic name for Alupent is metaproterenol. Albuterol is the generic name for Proventil and Ventolin. Isoetharine is the generic name for Bronkosol. Diphenhydramine is the generic name for Benadryl, which is not a drug administered by the EMT.

6.

D. Salmeterol xinafoate is the generic name for Serevent, a beta 2 specific agonist. Because it is a beta 2 agonist, it is prescribed to the patient, it is in a metered-dose inhaler, and the patient presents with the necessary indications, it is appropriate to assist the patient with the administration of the drug.

7.

C. Any time that you have a question about a treatment that involves medication administration, contact medical direction for clarification and further orders.

8.

D. All are true. The generic name is a shortened name assigned to the drug when it is approved by the FDA. The generic name is listed in the U.S. Pharmacopoeia. It also is commonly similar to the chemical name.

9.

A. An EMT ambulance carries oral glutose, an oral sugar medication used to treat hypoglycemic patients. The other three medications that are listed are typically not carried by the EMT ambulance; however, they are prescribed to the patient.

10.

B. Epinephrine is a drug that contains both alpha and beta properties. It is used to treat a patient suffering from an anaphylactic reaction. The alpha properties cause the vessels to constrict throughout the body. The beta 1 properties cause the heart rate to increase, the heart to contract more forcefully, and to speed the impulse down the conduction system, which are considered to be side effects from the drug administration. The beta 2 properties cause bronchiole smooth muscle relaxation. The EMT can assist the patient with epinephrine that comes in the form of an autoinjector.

11.

C. After assisting with the administration of any medication, it is important to recheck the patient for improvement or deterioration. This is achieved by conducting an ongoing assessment. Report any changes to medical direction and document these changes in the prehospital care report.

12.

B. The oral route is by mouth. The drug is swallowed and absorbed from the stomach or intestinal tract. Nitroglycerin is administered sublingually by either spray or tablet. If swallowed, the stomach acid and other contents render the drug ineffective.

Respiratory Emergencies

13.

C. Even though the diaphragm is a major muscle used in breathing, it lies outside the respiratory tract. The diaphragm separates the thoracic cavity from the abdominal cavity. It is found at the level of about the fifth intercostal space. The carina is the bifurcation of the trachea into the right and left mainstem bronchus. The larynx is the structure located superior to (above) the trachea. The bronchi are the main branches off of the trachea.

14.

D. Functions of the nose include warming, filtering, and humidifying inspired air.

15.

B. The epiglottis is a flap of cartilage that acts as a valve directing air into the trachea and food into the esophagus. The epiglottis prevents people from aspirating food and other substances into the trachea. When a person swallows, the larynx moves upward and the epiglottis moves downward, covering the glottic opening (opening into the larynx and eventually the trachea).

16.
C. The major muscle of respiration is the diaphragm. It contributes approximately 60 percent to 75 percent of the respiratory effort.

17.
A. A patient who is hypoxic can have a sympathetic response that causes an increase in the heart rate. A parasympathetic response causes the heart rate to decrease.

18.
D. An early sign of hypoxia is restlessness or agitation. Hypoxia causes the patient to become restless whereas the increasing levels of carbon dioxide in the blood (hypercarbia) cause the patient to become confused. Early during hypoxia, the skin becomes pale, cool, and clammy. Cyanosis is a late sign of hypoxia, and adults, children, and infants become tachycardic when hypoxic. Bradycardia is a very late and ominous sign of impending cardiac arrest, and the newborn initially becomes bradycardic when hypoxic.

19.
C. To determine whether the patient is breathing adequately, assess both the respiratory rate and tidal volume. To assess the tidal volume, inspect the chest rise with each ventilation. You must know both the respiratory rate and tidal volume before determining whether the patient is breathing adequately.

20.
C. Bilateral chest rise and fall with each ventilation indicate adequate ventilation. Cyanosis that turns gray can be a sign of worsened hypoxia. A patient who appears to be sleeping has a deteriorated mental status and could indicate a more severe hypoxic state. Upward abdominal movement with each ventilation can indicate a poor airway and excessive air movement into the stomach.

21.
B. The proportionate size of the tongue in an infant is larger than that of an adult.

22.
D. The narrowest portion of the upper airway in a patient under ten years of age is at the cricoid ring, which is below the vocal cords. The narrowest portion of an adult's airway is at the level of the vocal cords.

23.
B. The infant is exhibiting signs of a partial airway obstruction. The infant's stridorous respirations and color indicate that oxygenation/ventilation is still occurring. Allow the infant to continue to cough. Administer oxygen by nonrebreather mask or blow-by process. If a complete obstruction occurs, proceed to back blows and chest thrusts.

24.
C. If you suspect a partial airway obstruction, it is most important to keep your patient calm, instruct him to cough forcefully, and provide high-flow oxygen via a nonrebreather mask. If the patient deteriorates to a complete obstruction, immediately perform abdominal thrusts.

25.
A. In a complete airway obstruction, the patient is not able to cry or talk. In a partial airway obstruction, the patient coughs forcefully in an attempt to remove the object. If air is heard or felt on exhalation, the patient is still moving air and has a partial airway obstruction. Likewise, if breath sounds are still heard, the patient is still moving air in and out of the lungs, indicating a partial airway obstruction.

26.
A. Inspiration occurs due to the contraction of the diaphragm, causing it to move downward, and of the intercostal muscles, pulling the ribs outward, resulting in an increased thoracic cavity size, which causes the pressure within the thoracic

cavity to become negative, causing air to rush into the lungs to equalize the pressure.

27.
D. *Respiration* is the molecular process of exchanging oxygen and carbon dioxide. *Inspiration* is breathing in. *Ventilation* is the mechanical process of moving oxygen into the lungs and carbon dioxide out of the lungs. *Oxygenation* is the process of supplementing the oxygen content or providing oxygen therapy.

28.
D. The pharynx is a common passage way for food, water, and air.

29.
D. The occiput (back of the head) in the young child is disproportionately larger when compared with the child's body. The large occiput causes the flexion and leads to airway obstruction. To alleviate this problem in young children and infants, pad under the shoulders to bring the thorax up to the level of the head.

30.
D. The visceral pleura covers the lungs itself, becoming the outer most layer of the lungs, while the parietal pleura is in contact with the thoracic cavity. The peritonium is a lining in the abdominal cavity. The bronchioles are airway structures inside the lungs.

31.
D. The EMT must have protocol or online medical direction authorizing administration of a medication, and it must be prescribed to the patient. The EMT also must ensure that it is the right medication, right dose and right route and has not expired.

32.
D. The pharynx is divided into the oroparhynx and the nasopharynx. The larynx and the trachea are separate parts of the upper airway.

33.
C. The larynx, commonly referred to as the *voice box,* is a cartilaginous structure responsible for phonation.

34.
C. Do not administer the medication. The EMT can help administer medication only if it is prescribed for that patient. In this situation, explain your protocol to the family physician and defer further questioning to the medical director or on-line medical direction.

35.
D. Before helping with medication administration, the EMT must perform a thorough assessment to identify and manage any immediately life-threatening conditions.

36.
B. An indication of severe respiratory failure is a silent chest. The diminished breath sounds and decreased wheezing are caused by increasing bronchoconstriction and a severely decreased tidal volume. The patient is continuing to deteriorate and requires immediate intervention.

37.
B. When the EMT is performing positive pressure ventilation, the patient should have equal chest rise and fall, equal breath sounds bilaterally, and an improving mental status. A patient's pushing the mask away from his face during bag-valve-mask ventilation is a sign of an improving mental status. It does not mean that you can stop ventilating the patient, however. You must first reassess the patient to determine whether his respiratory rate and tidal volume are adequate enough to do so. A sign

of worsening hypoxia is a heart rate that continues to elevate. An increase in resistance when ventilating with a bag-valve-mask can indicate a poorly secured airway, an equipment malfunction, an upper or lower airway obstruction, or a developing pneumothorax.

38.

C. Stridor is caused by partial obstruction of the upper airway. Wheezing is caused by lower airway bronchiole constriction. Crackles or rales are due to fluid filled or collapsed terminal airways and alveoli.

39.

B. Asthma is a lower airway disease. Epiglottitis is a bacterial infection causing inflammation of the epiglottis and subglottic area in the upper airway.

40.

A. Patients who present in a tripod position (sitting upright and leaning forward, supporting themselves with their arms, with elbows locked between their dangling legs) are usually in respiratory distress. Occasionally, you can find a patient with severe respiratory distress lying supine or in a reclining position; these patients are usually so fatigued from the effort to breathe that they can no longer support themselves in an upright position. These patients appear very ill in the general impression.

41.

D. *Apnea* describes the condition of the patient who is in respiratory arrest. *Dyspnea* describes the patient who is having difficulty breathing. *Bradypnea* describes the patient who is breathing at a rate that is less than the normal. *Tachypnea* describes the patient breathing faster than the normal respiratory rate.

42.

B. Cyanosis is a bluish-gray skin color, which is an ominous sign of respiratory distress that requires immediate emergency care. Complaints of chest pain is not an indication that the patient is in respiratory distress; however, he is likely suffering from

an acute coronary syndrome. The patient who can speak only one or two words between breaths is in severe respiratory distress. Normal respiratory rates for children are 15 to 30/minute. It is normal for infants to use their abdominal muscles when breathing because their chest wall muscles are immature and are not used effectively.

43.

D. Stridor is a high-pitched inspiratory sound caused by a narrowing of the upper airway. Stridor indicates that the airway is partially obstructed by a foreign body or the swelling of the larynx.

44.

C. Hypotension (low blood pressure) is a late sign of respiratory distress in infants and children. A patient in respiratory failure requires immediate positive pressure ventilation. All other signs are seen in respiratory distress.

45.

B. Shallow chest rise is an indication that the patient has an inadequate tidal volume, which indicates inadequate breathing and requires positive pressure ventilation. Supplemental oxygen is connected to the bag-valve-mask device. Use of a non-rebreather mask alone is an ineffective treatment because of the inadequate tidal volume. The oxygen will remain in the dead air space and not reach the alveoli where the gas exchange is taking place. Even though this patient has an altered mental status, he would not be placed in a lateral recumbent position for two reasons: (1) he has suffered a head injury and the spine must be protected and (2) he requires ventilation, which cannot be provided in a lateral recumbent position. If ventilation is required, placing the patient in a supine position for ventilation is more important than placing him in a lateral recumbent position for drainage of fluids from the mouth.

46.

B. The airway is open and the respiratory rate and tidal volume are both adequate. Although the patient has an SpO2 of 94%, she is complaining of shortness of breath; therefore, you should provide supplemental oxygen by a nasal cannula.

47.

A. Loss of muscle tone is a sign of respiratory failure in an infant. The condition of respiratory failure is self-explanatory: the respiratory system has failed and can no longer provide adequate ventilation for the patient. Any patient who has signs of respiratory failure must be immediately ventilated. When you are ventilating, be sure that you are also providing supplemental oxygen through the ventilation device. Cyanosis around the nose and mouth is refered to as *circumoral cyanosis;* it is a sign of respiratory distress. Tachycardia (rapid heart rate) is a sign of respiratory distress, whereas bradycardia (slow heart rate) is a sign of respiratory failure in the infant. Prolonged exhalation and nasal flaring are early signs of breathing difficulty.

48.

B. If the child will not tolerate a nonrebreather mask, you should have the parent hold the child and administer oxygen using a blow-by method by holding the mask near but not on the child's face. Never withhold oxygen from any patient complaining of difficulty breathing. You should always speak to children softly; however, holding the mask on a child's face only adds to his stress and increases his work to breathe. Always reassure your patient. Administering oxygen by nasal cannula at 2 lpm is too low and not appropriate in this situation. Also, the patient does not have to breathe only through the nsoe when a nasal cannula is in place. When a nasal cannula is used, the oxygen collects in the nasopharynx and is drawn into the airway regardless of whether the patient breathes through his mouth or nose.

49.

C. Suspect that the child has epiglottitis if he has a fever, sore throat, is sitting upright with his neck jutted out, and drooling. Epiglottitis causes the epiglottis to swell and the larynx to spasm, blocking the opening into the trachea, is a true emergency, and should be treated with high-flow oxygen and immediate transport to the hospital. The condition has become much more rare due to vaccinating children for influenza. Any manipulation of the upper airway can cause laryngospasm (vocal cords spasm and close shut, not allowing any air to pass into the trachea) and lead to a complete upper airway obstruction. Even though the patient has a decreased tidal volume, this is one situation in which you would not aggravate the patient who is still moving air by inserting an airway or ventilation device. Apply a nonrebreather mask and maximize oxygenation. You should consider advanced life support backup.

50.

A. The action of the aerosolized medication in a metered-dose inhaler is a beta agonist, which relaxes the smooth muscle that lines the bronchioles. This drug, when administered, is inhaled and must travel deep into the lower airway where it is deposited on receptor sites on the bronchiole mucous lining. The beta agonist relaxes the smooth muscle and dilates the airway, relieving the bronchoconstriction and reducing the airway resistance.

51.

B. Do not administer a metered-dose inhaler (MDI) if the patient is not responsive enough to verbal stimuli to use the device. The MDI is effective only if the patient is able to take a deep breath to allow for the deposition of the particles deep in the respiratory tract.

52.

C. You should instruct the patient to inhale slowly and deeply over about 5 seconds as you or the patient depresses the canister. After has she inhaled the drug, you should coach her to attempt to hold her breath for 10 seconds. After doing so you should instruct her to exhale slowly through pursed lips.

53.

D. Ipratropium bromide (Atrovent®) is not a beta agonist and does not provide immediate action when inhaled. The EMT should not administer this drug. The other drugs are common beta agonists that are supplied in a metered-dose inhaler and can be given by the EMT after obtaining orders from medical direction.

54.

A. Tachycardia, tremors, shakiness, nervousness, dry mouth, nausea, and vomiting are all common side effects of the drug. Continue to reassess the patient while you look for signs of improvement or deterioration.

55.

A. The barking seal sound when the patient coughs is the hallmark of croup, which results in the swelling of the larynx, trachea, and bronchi. It is common for the condition to worsen at night. Apply oxygen, humidified if possible.

56.

A. Audible wheezes with diminished breath sounds are signs and symptoms of lower airway disease, such as asthma. A cough that produces a sound like a barking seal indicates croup, which is an upper airway problem. Fever with stridorous airway sounds and drooling are signs of epiglottitis, which occurs in the upper airway. Stridorous airway sounds that come on suddenly without other signs of sickness are likely from a partially blocked airway from a foreign body.

57.

C. The wheezing heard upon auscultation of breath sounds should lead you to suspect lower airway disease. This patient has been prescribed medication, which is delivered through a metered-dose inhaler. Knowing that Proventil® is a beta agonist that relaxes the bronchiole smooth muscle, you highly suspect that the child has a lower airway disease that results in bronchoconstriction. The condition the six-year-old child most likely has is asthma. Emphysema is also a lower airway disease; however,

it is found in adult patients. Epiglottitis and croup are both upper airway conditions.

Cardiovascular Emergencies

58.

A. Blood is pumped from the right atrium to the right ventricle and then into the pulmonary arteries where it is carried to the lungs for oxygenation. It leaves the pulmonary circulation and enters the pulmonary veins where it is carried back to the left atrium and then to the left ventricle. The blood is ejected from the left ventricle into the aorta and out to the systemic circulation throughout the body by the arteries.

59.

B. Oxygen, carbon dioxide, and other nutrients are exchanged between the cells and the blood in the capillaries.

60.

C. The right side of the heart is a low-pressure pump that pumps the blood through the pulmonary arteries to the lungs, which is a very low-pressure system. The left side of the heart is a high-pressure pump that must pump blood against the higher pressure found in the aorta and arteries throughout the body.

61.

D. The automated external defibrillator should be applied to patients who are unresponsive, pulseless, and have no breathing or abnormal breathing. This patient has agonal breathing, which is considered abnormal. Agonal breathing may occur in cardiac arrest patients. The AED can be applied to patients of all ages, including infants if necessary. In pediatric patients, it is preferred to use an AED with a pediatric attenuator device.

62.

C. A patient who is having difficulty breathing should be placed with the head of the cot in a Fowler's position, which is upright with the head and chest in an elevated position and is typically the most comfortable position. Supine positioning usually makes the patient feel that it is more difficult to breathe.

63.

C. Ventricular fibrillation is the most common presenting rhythm in the first 8 minutes after cardiac arrest. As the heart becomes more acidotic, hypoxic, and loses its supply of nutrients, the rhythm likely deteriorates into asystole. Ventricular fibrillation is the rhythm that is most likely to be converted to a perfusing rhythm.

64.

C. Defibrillation is the most effective treatment to terminate ventricular fibrillation. Recent research has shown that patients who have suffered cardiac arrest prior to the arrival of an EMT need CPR to provide the heart the necessary oxygen and glucose to allow the defibrillation to be more successful. It is recommended that up to 3 minutes of CPR be performed before defibrillation if the cardiac arrest is not witnessed. CPR increases the chance of a successful conversion to a perfusing rhythm; however, the defibrillation converts the ventricular fibrillation rhythm.

65.

B. Prehospital ALS is an important link in the chain of survival. Patients need to receive definitive care that ALS units in the field can provide.

66.

D. The semiautomatic defibrillator requires the operator to turn the unit on and push a button to deliver a shock. The automatic defibrillator requires the EMT only to push the "on" button; the defibrillator assesses and defibrillates when necessary without any operator intervention. No one should ever be in contact with the patient during the defibrillation.

67.

D. The American Heart Association ECC 2005 standards recommend that only one defibrillation be delivered to the patient followed by five cycles of CPR. The three-stacked shock sequence is no longer recommended.

68.

D. You have witnessed the patient's cardiac arrest and you have verified that he is unresponsive, pulseless, and apneic, so you should immediately attach the defibrillator and deliver a shock if indicated. If you do not witness the cardiac arrest, perform five cycles of CPR (approximately 2 minutes) and then attach the defibrillator and shock if advised.

69.

C. Defibrillation has been proven to be the most effective treatment for ventricular fibrillation. Reducing the time to defibrillation, working with advanced life support units effectively, and determining whether further training is needed are all aspects of the defibrillation that can be reviewed.

70.

B. If the cardiac arrest is not witnessed, you should perform five cycles of CPR (approximately 2 minutes) beginning with chest compressions. During the CPR, attach the defibrillator pads with minimal interruptions to chest compressions. Turn on the device for analysis after the fifth cycle and shock if advised.

71.

A. After delivering the first defibrillation, resume chest compressions immediately. The CPR sequence begins with the chest compressions, not ventilation, to restore perfusion pressures as quickly as possible. Complete five cycles of CPR before again analyzing the rhythm.

72.

D. Weak or dead batteries are the most common cause of the failure. Because of this, it is imperative to check the batteries before each shift.

73.

C. The operator checklist should be completed at the beginning of each shift or at least once per day. Completing the checklist ensures that the automated external defibrillator is in proper working order and that all of its necessary components are present and in working order.

74.
D. Studies have shown that to be most effective, the defibrillation should occur following five cycles (approximately 2 minutes) of CPR. This allows the necessary oxygen and nutrients to reach the heart and increase the success of conversion.

75.
A. The studies have shown that if bystander CPR is started immediately and defibrillation is done within 5 minutes following sudden cardiac arrest, the patient has the best chance of surviving with intact neurologic function.

76.
D. CPR should be performed after the first shock for five cycles followed by analysis of the patient's rhythm.

77.
C. Once a defibrillation has been delivered, the next immediate action is to begin chest compressions, even before checking pulses. Chest compressions are indicated immediately after the defibrillation if a nonshockable rhythm is detected. Chest compressions are begun first to increase the perfusion pressures and improve circulation to the brain, heart, and other vital organs.

78.
C. The automated external defibrillator should be placed only on an unresponsive, pulseless, and apneic patient. The hypoglycemic patient who is in cardiac arrest can benefit from defibrillation. A major risk factor for coronary artery disease is diabetes. Defibrillation rarely benefits patients in cardiac arrest from a traumatic incident, especially patients who have suffered a head injury.

79.
B. When two rescuers are present, one can prepare the defibrillator and place it on the patient's chest while the other performs five cycles of CPR prior to delivering the first defibrillation.

80.
D. A single rescuer needs to take the necessary body substance isolation precautions; determine whether the patient is unresponsive, apneic, and pulseless; do five cycles of CPR; apply the automated external defibrillator, and analyze the rhythm.

81.
A. If the patient becomes pulseless and apneic, it may be necessary to pull the ambulance off the road for safety purposes and to get additional assistance from the driver if it is only a two-person crew. Because the cardiac arrest is witnessed, defibrillation is most likely to be successful within the first few minutes. Thus, analyze the patient's rhythm and provide a defibrillation if indicated, immediately followed by chest compressions.

82.
B. This situation is a witnessed cardiac arrest, and the patient needs to be defibrillated immediately. Do not delay defibrillation for CPR, ventilation, or transport. One defibrillation should be delivered, followed by CPR.

83.
C. The postresuscitation patient should be reassessed at least every 5 minutes or immediately if his condition changes.

84.
B. The fully automatic defibrillator analyzes the rhythm and delivers the defibrillation without the operator having to manually press a button.

85.
D. The key element to successful defibrillation is the length of time before it is performed. The shorter the period of time before defibrillation, the more likely it is to be successful. The time is a

critical piece of information to document in your prehospital care report.

86.
C. When you are ordered to perform a procedure outside your protocol, report this and revert to the standing orders and/or contact medical direction for advice.

87.
D. To reduce anxiety, which could help reduce the chest pain, the patient should be placed in the position he feels most comfortable in. Never force a patient into a position in which he does not feel comfortable

88.
B. The batteries in an automated external defibrillator should be checked every day to prevent failure.

89.
C. When the automated external defibrillator advises "No Shock," immediately begin chest compression and perform CPR for five cycles before reassessing for a pulse and reanalyzing the rhythm.

90.
D. The automated external defibrillator should be used only with an unresponsive, pulseless, apneic patient. Pediatric defibrillation pads, which deliver a reduced amount of energy to the patient, should be used in patients who are a pre-puberty age. If the patient has an automated implanted cardiac defibrillator, defibrillation can still be done in a normal order without any harm to the patient. Avoid placing the AED pads over the implanted device.

91.
C. The proper sequence of events is to take body substance isolation precautions; determine unresponsiveness, pulselessness, and apnea; have your partner initiate CPR beginning with chest compressions, and perform five cycles while you prepare the AED; attach the AED; initiate the rhythm analysis after the five cycles of CPR; and deliver a defibrillation if indicated.

92.
A. The EMT must determine the systolic blood pressure, which should be at or above 100 mmHg, before administering a second or subsequent dose. Perform an ongoing assessment to determine whether the nitroglycerin has had an effect by assessing whether any relief of the chest pain or chest discomfort has occurred.

93.
D. The right side of the heart receives oxygen-depleted blood from the views and pumps oxygenated blood to the lungs and finally into the left side of the heart to be circulated throughout the body.

94.
C. Oxygen is no longer routinely administered at 15 lpm by nonrebreather mask in suspected acute coronary syndrome patients. If the patient has an SpO2 reading less than 94%; complains of dyspnea; or exhibits signs or symptoms of shock, hypoxia, or heart failure, oxygen should be administered. Begin with a nasal cannula at 2 to 4 lpm and titrate until the SpO2 reaches 94% or greater and the signs and symptoms are eliminated. If the patient continues to deteriorate or worsen, switch to a nonrebreather mask at 15 lpm.

95.
D. Although the SpO2 reading is above 94%, you should provide supplemental oxygen because the patient is complaining of shortness of breath. Begin with a nasal cannula at 2 to 4 lpm. You should place the patient in the position in which he is most comfortable. This helps reduce anxiety.

96.
D. The patient has a respiratory rate of 12/minute; however, the depth is shallow, indicating an inadequate tidal volume. Even though the rate is adequate, the shallow tidal volume indicates inadequate breathing, which requires ventilating the

patient. Placing the patient on a nonrebreather mask would not improve the breathing status because the tidal volume is inadequate and the shallow breaths will not likely transport the oxygen to the alveoli. Unrespon-sive patients should be placed in a lateral recumbent position; however, this patient requires ventilation, which cannot be done with the patient on his side. The patient who requires ventilation must be placed in a supine position, which takes precedence over placing him in a lateral recumbent position. An oropharyngeal airway is an airway adjunct that does not manage the patient's poor ventilation status.

97.
A. Approximately 20 percent of heart attacks are "silent"; that is, no chest pain is associated with the event. Silent heart attacks occur more frequently in elderly patients who have diabetics because of their diminished sensation of pain. Other assessment findings such as shortness of breath, nausea, vomiting, anxiety, abnormal blood pressure, abnormal pulse, dizziness, and feeling of impending doom should raise your suspicion of a silent heart attack.

98.
B. Nitroglycerin spray is administered sublingually as are the tablets. *Sublingual* refers to under the tongue; medication in the form of a spray or tablet, which is then absorbed into the blood stream. Nitroglycerin paste is administered through the skin but is not considered appropriate for the EMT to administer. Nitroglycerin can also be administered by intravenous drip but by hospital personnel and paramedics.

99.
A. This patient's blood pressure is 98/52 mmHg, which is too low to administer nitroglycerin. You should not administer nitroglycerin to patients with a systolic blood pressure of less than 100 mmHg. Other contraindications include patients with a suspected head injury and these who have already taken more than three doses as well as infants and children.

100.
B. Blurred vision, abdominal pain, or increased systolic blood pressure are *not* common side effects of nitroglycerin. Because nitroglycerin dilates blood vessels, the patient could experience a headache, a decrease in the blood pressure (hypotension), and a reflexive tachycardia.

101.
A. Because the patient is complaining of chest discomfort, shortness of breath, and nausea, it is likely that he is alert, has an adequate airway, and adequate breathing. The next step in the initial assessment is to assess circulation which includes the pulse and skin.

102.
C. The links in the 2010 American Heart Association Guidelines for Cardiopulmonary Resuscitation and Emergency Cardiovascular Care are immediate recognition and activation, early CPR, rapid defibrillation, effective advanced life support, and integrated post-cardiac arrest care. Early access is crucial. The sooner CPR is provided, the better are the chances for the patient's survival. Early defibrillation can restore a functional heartbeat to the patient, thus providing better circulation of oxygen. Effective advanced life support will provide medications and other techniques that increase the survival of the patient and reduce the chance of the patient refibrillating. Post-cardiac arrest care is essential for patient stabilization and resuscitating the brain. Early diagnosis, cardiac pacing, and intravenous therapy are not a part of the chain of survival.

103.
D. Ventricular fibrillation quickly degenerates into asystole (no electrical activity in the heart or "flat line"). The most effective defibrillation with successful conversion typically occurs within 4 minutes of the onset of cardiac arrest. As time elapses without defibrillation, the success rate falls significantly.

104.
C. Your goal as an EMT is to minimize the time from delivery of automated external defibrillation shocks to the arrival of advanced cardiac life support. If a paramedic unit is not available to respond to the scene or meet with your unit while you are en route to the hospital, you should continue with CPR and defibrillation. Remember early that advanced life support is a link in the chain of survival.

105.
D. The correct placement of the defibrillator pads is (−) on the right upper border of the sternum, and with the top of the (−) just below the clavicle. The (+) pad is placed over the left lower ribs at the left anterior axillary line. An alternative placement is anterior and posterior with the (−) posterior near the center of the back and the (+) anterior over the apex of the heart.

106.
A. Following a defibrillation, you must immediately begin chest compressions. Although the shock may have been successful and the patient has regained a pulse, two minutes of CPR will not harm the patient and may assist the heart with circulating the blood.

107.
C. The semiautomated and fully automated defibrillators are very similar; however, the fully automated device automatically delivers a shock if it senses that one is appropriate. An AED should not be used on children under the age of one year. Neither fully automated, nor semiautomated devices can effectively analyze the rhythm during CPR. Both types recognize asystole and will *not* deliver a shock in this case.

108.
D. The automated external defibrillator (AED) cannot effectively analyze the rhythm during CPR. The compression of the heart muscle produces electrical activity that produces artifact. The AED reads this rhythm and is unable to determine whether a shock is needed. The semiautomated defibrillator delivers a shock only when the EMT presses the button.

109.
B. Manual defibrillators require the use of paddles that must be held against the patient's chest. The AED uses external adhesive pads that attach to the patient and deliver a "hands-free" shock, which is considered safer for EMS personnel although it can shock the personnel if someone is touching the patient when the shock is delivered. The AED produces the same amount of energy as the manual defibrillators. Do not use the device while either you, the patient, or the device is wet. Dry yourself, the patient and the device after you have moved to a dry environment.

110.
D. The AED is a sensitive device that can be influenced by outside interference. When it is analyzing the patient between shocks, you should not touch the patient. Touching could interfere with the analysis.

111.
A. When using an older model monophasic AED during transport, you must stop the ambulance and turn the motor off. The older model AED can pick up the vibration from the motor, which interferes with the analysis of the rhythm.

112.
B. Interior lights of a vehicle are not likely to interfere with the automated external defibrillator analysis of the rhythm. The automated external defibrillator (AED) is a sensitive instrument; therefore, moving the patient can interfere with its analysis of the rhythm. Vehicle engine interference can increase the likelihood of the AED's false interpretation of the patient's rhythm.

113.
B. Your next action after checking the pulse following successful defibrillation is to assess the patient's breathing status. If breathing is adequate (rate and tidal volume), provide oxygen at 15 lpm via a nonrebreather mask. If the breathing is inadequate,

provide positive pressure ventilation with supplemental oxygen by bag-valve mask or another ventilation device.

114.
B. Most AED failures are the result of poor maintenance, especially of the battery. The AED and its batteries should be serviced on a regular schedule. Always check the AED at the beginning of every shift and carry extra charged batteries.

115.
A. High concentration oxygen is no longer routinely administered to patients. Administer oxygen in suspected acute coronary syndrome patients if the SpO2 is <94%, the patient complains of dyspnea, or signs and symptoms of shock, heart failure, or hypoxia are present. The pale, cool skin may be an early indication of hypoxia in this patient; therefore, administer supplemental oxygen via a nasal cannula at 2 to 4 lpm.

116.
A. Placing the patient in a position of comfort reduces anxiety and stress. Let the patient dictate the position that is most comfortable for him.

117.
C. You should reassure the patient that these changes are common side effects of the drug. It is unlikely that the patient is sensitive to this drug. Signs of anaphylaxis are itching, hives, redness, and increased difficulty breathing. Do not administer another nitroglycerin tablet until you reassess the patient's vital signs.

118.
B. The AED can be used on patients of any age. A pediatric dose attenuator should be used on pediatric patients if available. If not available, the adult AED should be applied, even to the infant. An unresponsive patient with no signs of life is an indication for CPR and application of the AED. It is not typically indicated for the patient in cardiac arrest resulting from trauma.

119.
D. Pediatric pads should be used in patients between one and eight years of age. If pediatric pads are not available, proceed by attaching the adult AED pads.

120.
A. Patients suffering from cardiac emergencies fall into two general categories: unresponsive in cardiac arrest and responsive with chest discomfort.

121.
C. All patients with chest pain do not go into cardiac arrest, but they can do so. Monitor the chest pain patient closely. If he becomes unresponsive, pulseless, and breathless, apply the AED.

122.
C. The fully automatic defibrillator requires the operator to push a single "on" button and the device does the rest. It analyzes the rhythm, determines whether ventricular fibrillation (or pulseless ventricular tachycardia) is present and then if it is, delivers the shocks. The semiautomatic defibrillator requires the operator to turn the unit on, possibly push a button to analyze the rhythm, and then push a button to provide a shock.

123.
A. The defibrillation could disrupt the hearts conduction system and cause a lethal dysrhythmia to occur. Prevent the administration of an inappropriate defibrillation to a patient by ensuring that he is unresponsive, pulseless, and breathless before attaching the device. A patient's heart can be damaged by the inappropriate administration of a defibrillation.

124.
C. The AED does not require the EMT to place his hands near the patient's chest during the defibrillation, lessening the chances of inadvertently shocking him.

125.

B. The AED is used to treat ventricular tachycardia without a pulse and ventricular fibrillation.

126.

C. If advanced life support is unavailable, the patient should be transported when the AED has given three consecutive "No Shock" messages or when one of the following occurs: (1) the patient's pulse returns or (2) a total of three individual shocks have been delivered.

127.

C. To increase the chance of successfully resuscitating a cardiac arrest patient in the prehospital setting, it requires all of the items in the chain of survival to be present. However, the only way to successfully and directly terminate ventricular fibrillation is by rapid defibrillation. The other items can improve the chance of successfully terminating ventricular fibrillation, but without defibrillation, the rhythm will continue regardless of performing the other items in the chain.

128.

C. Frequent practice ensures that the EMT can properly apply and operate the device. Practice also ensures that the EMT can properly recognize when the device is needed.

129.

C. Medical direction is responsible for all aspects of the use of defibrillators by EMS, who utilize them under the medical director's control. Defibrillation is the most effective method to terminate ventricular fibrillation; there is no alternative. Time is a critical factor that must be considered when implementing defibrillation programs and performing quality assurance/quality improvement audits. Allowing only ALS units to respond to cardiac arrest calls would likely delay the time to defibrillation and decrease the success rate of resuscitation. The use of EMT units that are closer and respond more quickly to provide defibrillation is a necessary consideration in successful defibrillation programs.

130.

A. Medical direction for the program must be involved in the audit process. Medical direction or a designated representative should review all incidents in which AED uses. These reviews could identify potential areas requiring improvement. Waiting to establish online medical direction delays the time to defibrillation, the critical factor to the successful termination of ventricular fibrillation.

131.

C. Defibrillation or the use of an automated external defibrillator (AED) is most useful for patients in cardiac arrest resulting from dysrhythmias associated with coronary artery disease. Ischemic stroke and hypoglycemic patients rarely present in cardiac arrest. Attaching the AED to patients with traumatic cardiac arrest is not a priority because they are likely not in ventricular fibrillation or the cause of the cardiac arrest is not due to a dysrhythmia or coronary artery disease.

132.

D. When applying an automated external defibrillator to a child who is between one and eight years of age, pediatric pads and cables should be used. The pediatric cables reduce the amount of energy delivered to the pediatric patient. If no pediatric pads and cables are available, proceed by attaching the adult pads and cables.

133.

C. Nitroglycerin can lower a patient's blood pressure. For this reason, it is contraindicated if the patient's systolic blood pressure is less than 100 mmHg.

134.

B. Nitroglycerin should be administered to a total of three doses. Recheck the blood pressure after each dose to ensure that the systolic blood pressure remains at 100 mmHg or higher. If the systolic blood pressure drops below 100 mmHg, stop administering nitroglycerin and continue to reassess the patient.

135.

D. Nitroglycerin dilates the blood vessels not only in the heart but also in other parts of the body, including the cerebral vessels. This dilation causes an increase in blood volume in the cranium, increasing the pressure and commonly causing the complaint of a headache.

136.

D. Automated and semiautomated external defibrillators are equally effective, and the AHA has endorsed both as being safe and effective. It is easier to learn how to operate an AED than it is to learn CPR. AEDs are able to detect loose leads or false readings of the EKG.

137.

D. All three signs of cardiac arrest—no respirations, no pulse, and response to painful stimuli (unresponsive)—must be present to apply the AED. If the radial pulses are absent, it is necessary to immediately assess the carotid pulse to determine whether the patient actually has or does not have a pulse.

138.

D. If ALS backup has been delayed, you should continue to treat the patient in most circumstances and transport him immediately after regaining a pulse. Do not remove the AED from the patient in the prehospital setting after it has been applied.

139.

D. The patient has reached the maximum of three total doses of nitroglycerin. Additional doses should be administered only after consulting medical direction. After three doses of nitroglycerin with no relief, you should suspect that the patient is having a myocardial infarction. If your orders allow, administer 325 mg of aspirin to the patient.

140.

B. If it advises "No Shock," immediately begin chest compressions. Perform five cycles of CPR and then reanalyze the rhythm.

141.

C. Ensure that all rescuers and bystanders are clear of the patient.

Diabetes/Altered Mental Status

142.

C. The patient is exhibiting the common signs of hypoglycemia: altered mental status; pale, cool, clammy skin; and tachycardia. Micronase is an oral hypoglycemia agent that Type II diabetes mellitus patients take. Based on the findings, the patient is exhibiting signs of hypoglycemia.

143.

D. A patient suffering from hypoglycemia exhibits a rapid onset of signs and symptoms: pale, cool, and clammy skin; an altered mental status due to the glucose deficiency; and tachycardia.

144.

A. A patient must have an intact gag reflex and the ability to swallow to receive instant oral glucose.

145.

C. The glucose should be placed on a tongue depressor and deposited between the gum and the cheek to dissolve in the patient's mouth. Rubbing the area can increase the absorption rate.

146.

D. The patient has an altered mental status and a partially occluded airway evident by the sonorous (snoring) airway sounds. The first priority in the initial assessment is to open the airway using a head-tilt, chin-lift maneuver because no trauma is suspected. After opening the airway, your next step is to assess the ventilation rate and tidal volume. You would then determine whether to apply a nonrebreather mask or to begin ventilation. Afterward, you would assess the pulse and skin. Oral glucose is not indicated because the patient is unresponsive.

147.

A. The patient who is unable to protect his own airway should not receive oral glucose.

148.

C. Your priority in managing the patient is to establish and maintain an open airway. You then should assess the ventilation status and determine the need to administer positive pressure ventilation or oxygen by nonrebreather mask at 15 lpm. Following the initial assessment, you would determine whether the patient has a gag reflex, is able to swallow, and is alert enough to receive oral glucose. It is necessary first to identify and manage all immediate life threats.

149.

B. An 8- to 12-hour fasting blood glucose level in a patient who is not diabetic should be around 80 to 90 mg/dL. If the patient has a history of diabetes, the fasting blood glucose level is often around 120 to 130 mg/dL. The glucose level of a nondiabetic patient up to several hours after eating a meal is typically 120 to 140 mg/dL, whereas in the diabetic it is often higher than 200 mg/dL.

150.

D. The treatment for this patient is to maintain an open airway, administer high-flow oxygen, position the patient on his side, and transport him. The patient must meet three criteria before you administer oral glucose: (1) have an altered mental status, (2) have a history of diabetes controlled by medication, and (3) be alert enough to swallow. This patient responded only to tactile stimulation and would not be able to protect his own airway, so you should not administer oral glucose.

151.

B. There are two acceptable ways to administer oral glucose: (1) hold back the cheek and squeeze a small amount of glucose between the cheek and gum and (2) place a small portion onto a tongue depressor, pull back the cheek, and deposit the medication between the cheek and gum by sliding the depressor in place.

152.

A. If the patient becomes unresponsive while you are administering oral glucose, remove the tongue depressor and reassess the airway, breathing, and circulation. Placing the unresponsive patient in a Fowler's position can compromise the airway; placement should instead be in a lateral recumbent position. Do not try to remove the glucose from the patient's cheek. This is a small amount and will not likely compromise the airway. Do not administer additional glucose to the unresponsive patient because it is contraindicated in this situation.

153.

B. Airway maintenance is the priority of care in the patient experiencing an altered mental status. The next step is to maintain adequate ventilation and oxygenation.

154.

D. Assess, establish, and manage the airway, breathing, and circulation during the initial assessment. Because the patient is unresponsive, you would suction secretions, administer oxygen, do a rapid head-to-toe physical exam, and attempt to obtain a SAMPLE history.

155.

A. A patient who has an altered mental status and requires ventilation must be kept in a supine position. It is not possible to effectively ventilate a patient in any other position. If the patient does not require ventilation and there is no suspicion of a spine injury, place the patient in a lateral recumbent position.

156.

D. Oral glucose is contraindicated in patients who have suffered a head injury, stroke, or some other type of problem that affects the brain. Research has shown that glucose administration in these patients worsens the patient's neurologic outcome unless he has a confirmed low blood glucose level. Type I and II diabetics are the typical diabetic patients who tend to become hypoglycemic; hypoglycemia is higher for Type I diabetics than Type II diabetics. Too much insulin in the blood is the cause of hypoglycemia; thus, you would *not* withhold glucose for that purpose.

Stroke

157.

D. An ischemic stroke is caused by a blocked cerebral artery, a common sign of which is facial droop. Headache and vomiting is associated with a hemorrhagic stroke. Shortness of breath is not common to either type of stroke.

158.

C. The signs and symptoms of TIA, often called a "ministroke" and is often a predictor of an impending stroke, typically resolve within 1 hour after onset, but always within 24 hours and leave no permanent cognitive, temporary, sensory, or motor deficits. This is the only obvious difference between a TIA and a stroke. TIA patients must still be transported since a significant number of these patients will soon suffer a stroke.

159.

A. This patient is exhibiting classic signs and symptoms of a stroke. Your initial treatment should be to establish and maintain an airway, adequate ventilation, oxygenation and circulation. Because the SpO2 reading is 93%, apply a nasal cannula at 2 to 4 lpm.

160.

B. Hemorrhagic strokes are commonly associated with chronic hypertension and congenital defects in cerebral arteries. The severe headache is caused by the sudden increase in intracranial pressure associated with rupture of an artery and collection of blood within the brain tissue or skull.

161.

B. Emboli can be caused by placque or stagnant blood particles from the left side of the heart, carotid arteries, or cerebral circulation. The others listed would enter the venous system and end in the pulmonary circulation resulting in a pulmonary embolism. The most common condition associated with an ischemic stroke is atrial fibrillation during which the atria fibrillate, dilate, and cause the blood to stagnate, increasing the risk of clot development. The clot would then travel to the left ventricle where it would be ejected into the carotid artery to the brain or in the systemic circulation through the aorta.

162.

D. A stiff neck is often a late sign of stroke caused by hemorrhage. The other signs or symptoms commonly occur at the onset of the stroke.

163.

C. Severe intermittent abdominal pain is not a sign or symptom of stroke. *Hemiplegia* is the medical term used to describe one-sided paralysis. Loss of bowel and bladder control and vision disturbances are common stroke signs and symptoms.

164.

B. The time of the first onset of the signs and symptoms of a stroke is critical because the thrombolytic drugs (used to break up the clot) must be administered within 3 hours of onset of the first sign or symptom of ischemic stroke. Another critical indicator is the score from the Cincinnati Prehospital Stroke Scale (CPSS) or the Los Angeles Prehospital Stroke Screen (LAPSS), which is highly predictive in determining whether the patient has had a stroke.

Allergic Reactions and Anaphylaxis

165.

B. During an allergic reaction, the hypoxia and leakage of fluid out of the vessels result in an increased heart rate. *Urticaria* is hives, and *pruritis* is itching, the hallmarks of allergic reaction.

166.

D. During an allergic reaction, the release of histamine and chemical mediators cause edema of the airway, increased mucus production, bronchial smooth muscle constriction, dilation of vessels, and an increase in capillary permeability, causing the capillaries to leak fluid.

167.

A. This patient is exhibiting signs and symptoms of a severe allergic reaction or anaphylaxis. Aggressive airway management and ventilatory support are of primary concern. Contacting Advanced Life Support is important; however, you must manage the airway and ventilation.

168.

C. This patient is exhibiting signs of a mild reaction including the urticaria (hives) and pruritis (itching). This patient could advance to a more severe reaction within minutes, so constant reassessment of the airway, breathing, and circulation is necessary. Without respiratory or cardiovascular system involvement, there is no need to administer the epinephrine. Once it is evident that the respiratory system or cardiovascular system is involved, however, do not delay epinephrine administration.

169.

A. A mild reaction can rapidly deteriorate to severe anaphylaxis involving severe respiratory compromise and cardiovascular collapse. Always be prepared to manage a severe reaction in the patient. If the patient has an epinephrine autoinjector, always keep it with the patient.

170.

A. Hypotension indicates cardiovascular compromise and the immediate need for epinephrine administration. Tachycardia is a common sign even in a mild reaction. The tachycardia could be caused by the reaction or by the anxiety that the patient is experiencing. Likewise, urticaria (hives) and flushed skin are found in mild reactions.

171.

B. Anaphylactic shock is characterized by severe respiratory compromise and cardiovascular collapse, which can include hypoperfusion, decreased level of consciousness, bilateral wheezing in all lung fields, nasal flaring, and tachypnea.

172.

C. The high-pitched sounds are stridorous sounds heard on inhalation. Stridor indicates obstruction of the upper airway, usually from the swelling of the larynx. The swelling in anaphylaxis is due to leakage of fluid from the capillaries into the tissue. The patient needs rapid and aggressive airway provision.

173.

B. Skin signs are typically the first to appear in the anaphylactic patient who usually presents with hives and itching. The skin also becomes red or flushed.

174.

D. The use and the administration of the epinephrine by autoinjector requires either an off-line or on-line order from medical direction. The medication is prescribed to the patient by intramuscular injection.

175.

B. If the patient is suffering from a mild allergic reaction without respiratory compromise or signs of shock, do not administer epinephrine by autoinjector. Treatment includes administering high-flow oxygen, placing the patient in a position of comfort, completing your assessment, and transporting the patient. Aspirin is used only if the patient is suspected of having a myocardial infarction.

176.

A. You may need to force air past the swollen laryngeal tissue using the bag-valve-mask (BVM) unit by providing positive pressure ventilation. Delivering ventilation could become difficult due to the high resistance, but deactivating the BVM's pop-off valve can help deliver adequate ventilation. The airway is compromised due to swelling of laryngeal tissue; thus, inserting an airway adjunct, such as the OPA and NPA, are of little help.

177.

C. The correct administration for a prescribed epinephrine autoinjector is to (1) firmly push it against the patient's thigh midway between the knee and the waist and (2) hold it in place until all of the drug has been delivered. The injector delivers the correct dose automatically if it is left in place until it is empty.

178.

C. The possible side effects to the administration of epinephrine are headache, dizziness, chest pain, increased heart rate, pale skin, nausea, vomiting, and anxiousness. You should advise your patient of these possible side effects when you administer the drug.

179.

A. Administration of epinephrine by autoinjector in the severe anaphylactic patient has no contraindications. The autoinjector automatically delivers the adult a dose of 0.3 mg, so you should never deliver a half dose to any patient, although infants and children are prescribed epinephrine autoinjectors that deliver a dose of 0.15 mg. Stridorous respiration indicates that the anaphylactic patient's airway is becoming compromised, indicating the use of epinephrine by autoinjector.

Poisoning/Overdose Emergencies

180.

B. Patients with poisoning or an overdose can have dilated or constricted pupils; however, the pupils typically remain equal. Unequal pupils can indicate a brain injury from a stroke or trauma.

181.

D. Many patients who have overdosed on an unknown medication cannot maintain their airway, so your first concern is to open and maintain it. Positioning and using airway adjuncts such as the nasopharyngeal airway or the oropharyngeal airway could be necessary to maintain an open airway.

182.

B. You must immediately begin positive pressure ventilation because the respirations have deteriorated to an inadequate rate.

183.

C. A patient who has overdosed on blood pressure medication is a good candidate for activated charcoal, which can be used up to 4 hours after the ingestion of some medications. Activated charcoal is contraindicated in liquid bleach and ammonia. Activated charcoal is an adsorbent that is used for ingested poisonings, not inhalation.

184.
C. Activated charcoal is very porous; thus, it adsorbs the poison and inhibits its absorption by the body. Some poisons have slow absorption rates that allow activated charcoal to be used up to 4 hours after ingestion.

185.
D. The routes of entry into the human body include ingestion, inhalation, injection, and absorption. Typically, the fastest routes in which the poison enters the body is by injection and inhalation.

186.
C. Even though the medication is in a spray form, it is not inhaled but it is absorbed under the tongue in the very vascular oral mucosa, so it is referred to as *sublingual,* which means under the tongue.

187.
B. *Injection* is the mode of entry of a substance through a break in the skin. The break can be caused by a stinger, needle, or bite.

188.
C. Dry powders should be brushed off before the area is irrigated. Many chemicals are inactive in the powder form but are activated, or become more activated, when they come into contact with water, creating a reaction that increases the heat and extends the burn. Once the powder has been brushed off, irrigate the area with large amounts of water.

189.
D. The first priority for the EMT is always scene safety. The scene in this case is obviously unsafe because of the chlorine leak. The EMT's job is not the patients' extrication, which needs to be performed by trained personnel with specialized equipment.

190.
B. The patient should be placed in the lateral recumbent position to prevent the aspiration of secretions, vomitus, blood, and other substances.

191.
C. When you have a question concerning an overdose or toxicology, you should contact the local poison control center. It provides the most up-to-date information.

192.
A. All overdose patients should be transported to a medical facility to be seen by a physician because of the possible multiple problems. The drug or substance that the patient took or was exposed to may not have any severe effects until minutes to days after the exposure. Depending on the substance, the patient can appear fine but be unresponsive and unstable within several minutes.

193.
D. The patient needs immediate ventilation due to the excessive respiratory rate and inadequate tidal volume. An oropharyngeal airway should not be inserted because the drain cleaner has likely injured the oral tissue and insertion can aggravate it or cause further damage. The EMT should never give anything by mouth to a patient who has an altered level of consciousness who cannot protect his own airway. This would lead to the patient's aspiration of the substance.

194.
B. Establishing and maintaining a patent airway, performing a medical assessment, and administering oxygen are essential for the overdose patient. The administration of activated charcoal may or may not be indicated. It is contraindicated if the patient has an altered mental status or has swallowed bleach, ammonia, or hydrochloric acid. Some EMS systems have removed activated charcoal as a treatment choice.

195.
A. Activated charcoal is also known as Super-Char, InstaChar, Actidose, and Liqui-Char. Char-Med is not a trade name.

196.
A. Activated charcoal is useful for poisonings that occur only by ingestion.

197.
D. The contraindications for the use of activated charcoal include the patient who has an altered mental status, has swallowed acids or alkalis (hydrochloric acid, chlorine bleach, ammonia, ethanol), or is unable to swallow.

198.
B. Activated charcoal is available as a powder (not recommended for field use) and premixed in water. The premix bottle contains 12.5 grams of activated charcoal.

199.
A. The adult and child dose is 1 gram per kilogram of body weight. The usual dose for an adult is 25 to 50 grams and for a child it is 12.5 to 25 grams.

200.
D. Activated charcoal settles on the bottom of the container. For this reason, it should be shaken well or mixed prior to administration. It should never be administered without prior medical direction. Because of its appearance, the patient may be more willing to drink it if he cannot see it. Use an opaque container and have the patient drink through a straw if possible.

201.
A. Activated charcoal is extremely porous and adsorbs (binds to) poisons in the stomach and prevents absorption in the small intestine.

202.
C. The most common side effect of activated charcoal is a blackened stool. Nausea and vomiting may also occur, especially in a patient who is already nauseated. If the patient vomits after the administration of activated charcoal, contact medical direction and request permission to repeat the dose.

203.
D. Early contact with medical direction is required to obtain the most current treatment for a patient who has overdosed or ingested poison. Orders to administer activated charcoal are required. Early contact also allows the receiving facility to prepare for the patient's arrival.

204.
C. It is important to determine whether the patient is suffering from a medical condition or the effects of drugs and/or alcohol. Many medical conditions can mimic the effect of drugs and alcohol. Search the area immediately around the patient for evidence of drug or alcohol use. An unresponsive patient who has unequal pupils is likely suffering from a structural problem (head injury, stroke, tumor) within the cranium, not a drug- or alcohol-related problem. Open sores and scars to the upper arm can be associated with injection of drugs.

205.
A. Patients who have taken phencyclidine, or PCP, can become agitated and enraged if this technique is utilized. The "Talk-Down Technique" includes making the patient feel welcome, identifying yourself clearly, reassuring the patient, helping the patient verbalize what is taking place, repeating simple concrete statements, and explaining actions to be taken to the patient.

Environmental Emergencies

206.
D. The majority of heat lost through the human body is from the head, feet, and hands through radiation.

207.
C. Water conducts heat away from the human body 240 times faster than any other mechanism.

208.
B. Signs of early hypothermia include shivering, muscle stiffness, pale skin, and rapid heart rate. Bradycardia occurs later in hypothermia with more severe decreases in body core temperature.

209.
A. The core body temperature will drop 25 to 30 times faster because the body is in contact with cold water molecules. The body's temperature cools to the temperature of the ambient environment around it, in this case, the water temperature.

210.
C. Patients who are elderly typically have poor fluid intake and are commonly dehydrated, which predisposes them to heat emergencies. They also commonly suffer from poor thermoregulation. Some medications and pre-existing medical conditions also make them more prone to heat emergencies.

211.
A. The primary concern when managing a patient in heat stroke is to remove him from the hot environment to prevent his body from continuing to take on heat. The patient needs rapid cooling to prevent cellular breakdown due to the increased body temperature. You would never place the patient in ice or place ice on the patient because this will likely cause him to shiver, which increases the body core temperature. The patient should be kept in a supine or lateral recumbent position.

212.
D. Aspiration of salt water draws fluid into the interstitial space between the alveoli and the capillary and into the alveoli, leading to pulmonary edema. Auscultate the breath sounds for crackles/rales. Provide positive pressure ventilation and ensure that the ventilation device is connected and delivering high concentrations of oxygen.

213.
C. All patients who have been involved in a submersion incident or near drowning need to be transported and evaluated in the emergency department. Explain the consequences of pneumonia, pulmonary edema, respiratory failure, and even death to the patient.

214.
A. Infants and children suffer from heat emergencies because of their proportionately larger body surface areas, smaller body fat content, immature thermoregulatory centers, and the inability to dress or undress for the temperature exposure.

215.
B. Only one defibrillation should be provided if the patient is in cardiac arrest. A cold heart does not respond well to defibrillation or drug therapy. The severe hypothermic patient should be handled very gently to prevent ventricular fibrillation, which rough handling can cause. Do not rub or massage the patient's arms or legs because this could force cold venous blood into the core circulation and heart, resulting in cardiac arrest. If ventilation is required, avoid hyperventilation, which can cause further cardiac compromise and cool the patient faster if he is in a cold environment.

216.
C. If you are unable to obtain a pulse and there are no respirations but detect patient movement, delay CPR and the use of the automated external defibrillator. Pulses are very difficult to find in hypothermic patients. You should immediately begin positive pressure ventilation.

217.
B. The body temperature should be increased slowly. Add heat to the patient gradually and gently. The patient's body temperature should not be increased more than 1 degree fahrenheit per hour.

218.
B. Instruct the patient to remain as calm and immobile as possible with just enough effort to remain afloat. Lift the patient from the water in a horizontal or supine position. Remove the wet clothing as quickly and gently as possible to prevent further heat loss and ventricular fibrillation.

219.
B. Correct management includes the removal of jewelry. The tissue is likely to swell from the cold injury, and jewelry can create a tourniquet effect and cut off circulation to distal extremities. Avoid massaging the affected area and the application of salves or ointments. Blisters that are present should be left intact and should not be broken.

220.
D. Rewarming localized frozen tissue should generally be avoided unless you have a long or delayed transport. If you do rewarm, use water at 100 to 110 degrees Fahrenheit. Never use dry heat because its temperature is too difficult to control. Rewarming tissue is very painful, and medical direction commonly wants the patient to have an analgesic.

221.
C. Remove the stinger by scraping against it with the edge of a credit card or knife. Lower the injection site slightly below the level of the heart. Clean the site with a soap solution or a mild cleansing agent. The application of cold packs may help to reduce swelling at the injection site.

222.
D. Your first action should be to move the patient into the back of the air-conditioned ambulance. This is followed by removing the clothing, administering oxygen, and rapidly cooling the patient with a cool water spray and aggressive fanning.

223.
A. The patient most likely has heat stroke and requires rapid transport. Cooling should be continued en route to the hospital. Maintain an airway and monitor the respirations closely.

224.
D. Hot skin is an indication of a heat emergency, whereas dry skin is an indication that the patient is most likely dehydrated from excessive sweating prior to experiencing the heat stroke. Some heat stroke patients present with moist skin; however, it remains hot.

225.
A. Alcohol dilates blood vessels and interferes with the normal thermal regulatory mechanisms, which can increase the patient's risk of hypothermia. Family history is not a predisposing factor that increases the risk of hypothermia. A person's age is a major factor in the risk of hypothermia. The young and old are more likely to suffer from hypothermia, but middle-aged people are not more predisposed to it. Medical conditions such as head injury, spinal cord injury, stroke, diabetes, and a heart condition can increase the likelihood of hypothermia.

226.
C. Shivering is one of the body's first reactions to a decrease in body temperature found in the first stage of hypothermia. The second stage of hypothermia involves a decrease in fine and then gross motor function. The fine motor function decrease can be as subtle as the inability to follow simple commands. A decrease in the heart rate and respirations is the fourth stage of hypothermia. As the hypothermia continues, the patient might not be able to move his arms or legs.

227.
A. As long as the patient is responsive and not nauseated, administer a half glass of water every 15 minutes. This patient should be placed in a supine position with the feet elevated approximately 8 to 12 inches to increase the blood flow to the brain.

228.
B. You should lower the extremity below the level of the heart in an attempt to reduce the flow of venom to the systemic circulation. Cold packs should not be applied to the injection site of snakebites because cold packs can increase tissue damage at the injection site. Do not suck out the venom from the wound because this could envenomate you. Never apply a tourniquet to the extremity. A constricting band may be applied to reduce the venous blood flow.

229.
B. After stinging, bees tear their bodies from the stinger and the venom sack. This sack, if not removed, continues to pulsate, pumping venom into the patient. Remove the sack and stinger by scraping a knife or credit card edge against it. Squeezing the sack with tweezers or your fingers while attempting to remove it will force more venom from the sack into the patient. Never incise the patient for any reason.

230.
C. This patient's breathing is inadequate due to the extremely fast respiratory rate and poor tidal volume. You should immediately begin bag-valve-mask ventilation.

231.
A. You should immediately administer the epinephrine by autoinjector, but unless you have offline orders for the administration of epinephrine by autoinjector, you must obtain an online order before to administering it. Delaying this action could cause the patient's condition to deteriorate further. This patient is having a severe allergic reaction (anaphylaxis) and should receive epinephrine as quickly as possible.

232.
B. Common side effects of epinephrine are increased heart rate, pale skin, dizziness, chest pain, headache, nausea, vomiting, excitability, and anxiousness.

Psychiatric Emergencies

233.
B. A person's personality is just one aspect of his or her behavior. Depressions and anxiety are classifications of behaviors.

234.
C. Society has classified acceptable or "normal" behavior for many situations. Any deviation from the norms can be considered abnormal.

235.
D. Many different underlying causes produce these signs and symptoms, including head injury, oxygen deficits, altered glucose levels, and other deficiencies that could lead to abnormal behavior. Be sure to assess the patient carefully and check for an organic cause for the behavior.

236.
D. Patients who want to hurt themselves often use extreme measures to do so. Others can place themselves in high-risk situations. Report this information to the emergency department staff.

237.
C. A leading cause of suicide is depression over the loss of a loved one.

238.

B. Approximately 80 percent of patients who commit suicide made a failed previous attempt. This is one reason why all patients who have suicidal tendencies should be transported.

239.

C. The EMT should be concerned that the patient could have attempted suicide. You should directly ask the patient if he was attempting to kill himself.

240.

B. Patients who have constructed a plan on how to kill themselves are much more likely to carry out their intentions than are those who have no plan.

241.

B. When a patient informs you that he has thought of harming himself and has formulated a plan, you should become highly concerned for your safety and that of the patient, especially when a gun is involved in the plan. Reassess the scene safety and retreat if necessary.

242.

C. When any scene is unsafe, you should immediately remove yourself from it. Contact law enforcement to handle the weapon. When the scene is secure, enter it to manage the patient.

243.

B. Patients over the age of 40 are more likely to commit suicide. People who are elderly commonly suffer severe depression and are very likely to commit suicide. Depression in an elderly patient is considered a serious emergency.

244.

D. EMTs are most often injured when a patient's behavior changes rapidly. Patients who are intoxicated, under the influence of drugs, or have behavioral problems are most likely to have sudden behavior change. When assessing this type of patient, have adequate personnel to help restrain him if necessary. Make sure the scene is free from potential weapons and always have available exit routes. When responding to crime scenes, the perpetrators have typically fled the scene and are no longer a threat. Remember that scene safety never ends and the EMT is constantly assessing it.

245.

B. Any patient who is a suicide risk should never be left alone. Constant supervision is necessary to guarantee the safety of yourself and the patient.

246.

B. Many people who are incarcerated for crimes, some very minor, are likely to commit suicide due to the social impact on their reputation.

247.

D. All of the factors can cause aggression. Be sure not to rule out an organic cause.

248.

B. The job of the EMT is to be impartial, not judgmental. To assess whether the threat is real, you should ask the patient about his intention to kill himself, and how he would do it. The threat of suicide is higher when the plan is more realistic. Do not restrain suicide patients against their will unless they are definitely a threat to you.

249.

B. Once a patient has been restrained, leave the restraints on. The patient may be calm one minute and revert to the aggressive behavior the next.

Acute Abdominal Pain

250.

D. Patients suffering from acute abdominal pain try to stay completely still and quiet to decrease the pain. Drawing the knees to the chest releases some of the tension on the abdominal muscles and can slightly reduce the pain.

251.
B. The organs of the right upper quadrant include most of the liver, gallbladder, and part of the large intestine. The spleen and pancreas are located in the left upper quadrant.

252.
A. Irritation under the diaphragm can cause referred pain that can present as shoulder pain.

253.
B. The pulsatile mass, tearing pain radiating to the lower back, and the absent femoral pulses are signs indicative of an abdominal aneurysm that is currently rupturing. This is a dire emergency for which the treatment is to provide oxygen and rapid transport to an appropriate facility for emergency surgery.

254.
C. Cholecystitis or inflammation of the gallbladder is commonly precipitated by ingesting food high in saturated fat. The green vomitus is likely due to the obstruction of the bile duct.

255.
D. *Referred pain* is felt in a body part other than its point of origin. Pain associated with abdominal and other conditions can be referred or felt in other areas of the body. This phenomenon is associated with the proximity of separate nerve tracks as they enter the spinal cord.

256.
B. Common causes of abdominal pain include intestinal obstruction, pancreatitis, cholecystitis, hernia, ulcer, and abdominal aortic aneurysm.

257.
C. The correct position for a patient suffering from an acute abdominal pain with signs of hypoperfusion (shock) is supine with feet elevated. The patient should not be placed in a seated position due to the hypoperfusion state, which would cause a decrease in the blood flow to the brain.

258.
B. When treating a patient with acute abdominal pain without signs of hypoperfusion (shock), you should place the patient in the position of most comfort. Typically, patients with acute abdominal pain position themselves bent over at the waist with their knees bent and drawn up toward their chest. Often this position reduces the tension on the abdominal muscles, thus reducing pain.

259.
D. Allow the patient to assume a position of comfort and remain still. Never give a patient with acute abdominal pain anything by mouth. These patients need to be prepared to go to surgery if necessary, and the presence of food and liquid can cause vomiting after anesthesia administration, possibly leading to aspiration. Also, administration of milk or antacids can mask the patient's symptoms.

Obstetrics and Gynecology

260.
C. The uterus is a hollow muscle that houses the fetus until birth.

261.
B. The placenta is the organ that allows for gas exchange and nourishment of the fetus. The fetal lungs, gastrointestinal system, and liver are not functioning, so the placenta provides the necessary oxygen and nutrients and eliminates the carbon dioxide and other waste products.

262.
B. Contractions under 2 minutes and lasting 30 to 90 seconds, along with the patient's urgency to move her bowels (caused by the baby placing pressure on the rectum), are all signs that the baby is ready to deliver. However, you need to assess for crowning to determine how imminent the delivery is.

263.
C. The first clamp should be placed approximately 6 inches from the infant's abdomen.

264.
D. The birthing process involves many different body fluids, so the recommended body substance isolation precautions include mask, gown, gloves, and eye protection.

265.
B. The second clamp should be placed approximately 3 inches from the first clamp. You would then cut between the two clamps. It is extremely important to be sure there is no blood leaking from either end of the umbilical cord after it has been cut.

266.
D. If the neonate's respirations are depressed after drying him, you should next stimulate him by flicking the soles of his feet. If he still does not respond, you should then begin bag-valve-mask ventilation.

267.
C. If the infant's heart rate drops below 60 beats/minutes, chest compressions should be initiated.

268.
B. Meconium is fecal matter excreted by the infant, usually because of severe distress. Meconium

aspiration carries a high mortality rate. The EMT must recognize this problem and aggressively suction the airway to remove all evidence of meconium.

269.
C. Meconium is often present when the fetus becomes distressed from decreased oxygen level or a prolonged labor.

270.
D. Immediate suctioning of the infant's airway takes precedence over all other procedures to prevent aspiration of the meconium at all cost. Meconium aspiration could lead to severe respiratory depression.

271.
A. The *perineum* is the area of tissue between the vagina and anus. This area can tear during a rapid delivery or when the infant is large. The perineum is the area where the episiotomy is performed to facilitate delivery. When the head of the newborn is delivered, the EMT should gently place a gloved hand over the head to prevent an explosive delivery during a forceful contraction that could tear the perineum.

272.
B. The foul smell is from the meconium, and the airway needs to be suctioned immediately and aspiration prevented.

273.
D. Infants can respond quickly to short periods of ventilation. Once the ventilation is determined to be adequate, stop it and reassess.

274.
D. In one minute, 90 compressions and 30 ventilations are delivered in neonatal CPR. The ratio is three compressions to one ventilation.

275.
D. The correct depth is one-third the depth of the chest.

276.
A. Reassess the infant every 30 seconds to determine whether he is responding to the ventilation. The typical sequence in neonatal resuscitation is to intervene and continuously reassess.

277.
D. A condition that occurs during the third trimester of pregnancy, called *supine hypotensive syndrome,* occurs as a result of the combined weight of the fetus and uterus compressing the inferior vena cava. This pressure obstructs the blood return to the heart via the inferior vena cava while the patient is lying supine, causing hypotension. A common complaint is lightheadedness, dizziness, feeling faint, or actually suffering a syncopal episode (fainting) when the patient is in a supine position. You should place the patient on her left side or elevate the right hip to take the weight of the fetus and uterus off the vena cava and restore venous return to the heart.

278.
B. Cover the vaginal opening with a sanitary pad to collect the blood. Save and transport any passed tissue for examination by hospital personnel. Packing sanitary napkins or pads into the vagina is always inappropriate. If a pad becomes soaked with blood, it should be replaced. If bleeding is excessive, it can become a life-threatening emergency. Carefully evaluate the patient for signs and symptoms of shock.

279.
D. Delivery of a fetus before it is viable is a spontaneous abortion (miscarriage), which can occur for many different reasons. Viability is usually considered to begin after the 20th week of pregnancy. Signs and symptoms of spontaneous abortion include cramplike lower abdominal pain, moderate to severe vaginal bleeding, and passage of tissue or blood clots.

280.
D. Do not allow the mother to use the bathroom, even though she has the urge to defecate. This is likely a result of the infant's head moving down the birth canal and pressing against the patient's rectum. If you allow her to use the bathroom, she could deliver the neonate in the toilet.

281.
C. Recommended equipment for an obstetric kit includes surgical scissors, cord clamps or cord ties, umbilical tape, bulb syringe, towels, gauze sponges, sterile gloves, infant blanket, individually wrapped sanitary napkins, large plastic bag, and germicidal wipes. A bag-valve mask is not a part of the OB kit but is carried separately on the ambulance. It is a vital piece of equipment that must be available during the delivery of the neonate.

282.
B. As soon as the head is delivered, support it and suction the mouth first and then the nose. Compress the bulb syringe and suction two or three times to remove fluid and secretions. Insert the tip 1.0 to 1.5 inches into the infant's mouth. Avoid touching the back of the mouth with the tip of the bulb syringe.

283.
D. Excessive pressure should be avoided over the fontanel, or soft spot. Excessive pressure should not be used for any delivery procedure. Never grasp or apply pressure under the arms because this will likely result in severe nerve damage. The cord should be immediately removed from around the neck once it is found. If left in place, it could strangle the fetus as the delivery continues. If the amniotic sac is still intact when the head is delivered, immediately break the sac and remove it from the fetus' face.

284.
B. The EMT should check the position of the umbilical cord to determine whether it is wrapped around the infant's neck. The creation of a sterile field should have been accomplished prior to the delivery of the head. You will have plenty of time after delivery to record the time of birth.

285.
C. Up to 500 mL is normal. If blood loss is excessive, administer oxygen and provide uterine massage.

286.
D. Massage of the mother's uterus is provided to control excessive bleeding following delivery. Uterine massage helps to stimulate contractions and tone up the uterus, which reduces uterine size. This reduces bleeding.

287.
C. In multiple births (twins, triplets), the infants can either share a placenta or have separate ones.

288.
D. In multiple births, about one-third of all deliveries of the second infant is breech. A breech delivery is one in which the fetal buttocks or the lower extremities are the first to present in the birth canal.

289.
C. Ensuring the adequacy of the airway, breathing, and circulation always is a priority treatment for all patients. Oxygen administration is the next priority. This is followed by managing bleeding from the vagina. Transport is the last step.

290.
C. The pregnant trauma patient is able to compensate for blood loss because of an overall increase in body fluid. Late pregnancy patients are at greater risk for injuries to the uterus, liver, or spleen or rupture of the mother's diaphragm, even when the crash occurs at a relatively low speed. Potential fetal injuries can occur as well. In this case, the mother was unrestrained, so the potential for injury is present. The best answer presented is to recognize the compensatory capability of the pregnant patient. Encourage her to seek medical care and attention.

291.
D. Determining whether the patient has taken any over-the-counter medications is an appropriate question, just not as important as determining the pain characteristics. Evaluation of the quality of the pain allows you to determine whether the patient is experiencing labor pains or pain related to the accident.

292.
C. This patient should be evaluated for signs of crowning. The signs and symptoms presented can indicate immediate delivery. If the baby is crowning, prepare for delivery. The patient should not be placed in a supine position because of the possibility of supine hypotensive syndrome

293.
C. You should suction the mouth and nose of the infant as soon as the head is delivered and prior to delivery of the rest of the body. After the delivery of the torso, the newborn can breathe deeply because the chest is no longer being constricted in the birth canal. Suctioning the newborn's mouth and nose prior to delivery of the torso will help prevent it from aspirating the fluids in the mouth and nose.

294.
B. You should suction the mouth prior to suctioning the nose. Suctioning the mouth first prevents aspiration of fluid. Placing the bulb syringe and then compressing the bulb forces the fluid into the lungs. Advancing the tip of the bulb syringe too deeply into the pharynx can cause the newborn to become bradycardic. Suction the mouth and nose prior to stimulating the newborn to remove all secretions prior to spontaneous breathing.

295.

D. The pregnant patient who is near full term can experience supine hypotensive syndrome when lying on her back. To prevent this condition, elevate the right hip to shift the weight of the fetus and uterus off the inferior vena cava. If the patient feels comfortable, you can have her lie in a lateral position.

296.

D. Your first priority is to establish an airway by suctioning and positioning. A pregnant patient who is seizing could be experiencing eclampsia.

297.

D. You should avoid applying pressure to the infant's fontanel, the soft area on the infant's head. Gentle pressure can be applied horizontally to prevent an explosive delivery.

298.

A. When the placenta appears, grasp it and gently guide it from the vagina. Under no circumstances should you pull the placenta from the vagina or pull on the umbilical cord to try to deliver the placenta. Do not delay transport while waiting on delivery of the placenta. Do not dispose of the placenta but transport it to the hospital; the physician will need to examine it.

299.

A. The only time it is permissible to place your gloved hand into the mother's vagina is when you encounter a prolapsed cord. This presents a true emergency that can result in the infant's injury or death. When you encounter a prolapsed cord, you should insert your gloved hand into the vagina and gently push the presenting part away from the pulsating cord.

300.

A. The patient with a limb presentation should be placed in a supine position with the head lower than the rest of her body with the hips elevated. This position increases the gravity and slows the progress of the fetus through the birth canal. Administer oxygen and transport immediately. Never push or pull a presenting limb into the vagina. Never try to manipulate the fetus into the correct position by inserting your hand into the vagina. Cover the exposed limb with a moist sterile dressing.

301.

C. The infant born before the 38th week of pregnancy is considered premature. Infants weighing less than 5.5 pounds at birth are considered premature. The premature infant does not have cartilage in the outer ear. Premature babies appear smaller and skinnier than full-term infants and have red and wrinkled skin. Premature babies usually have a single crease across the soles of their feet. Premature infants have fine silky hair and very small breast nodules.

302.

B. This infant was born before the 38th week of gestation, which makes it premature. Premature infants need special care because their lungs and organs are not fully developed. Premature infants must be kept warm by using warmed blankets or a plastic bubble-bag swaddle. Never forcefully direct oxygen into the premature infant's face; hold the end of the oxygen tubing approximately .5 inch above the infant's mouth and nose. You should suction secretions gently, using the bulb syringe. To prevent heat loss, cover the premature infant's head, leaving the face exposed.

303.

B. Place this patient in a supine position with her hips elevated. This position helps to keep the fetus from putting pressure on the cord. All of the other positions listed can increase pressure on the cord.

304.

A. You should place your gloved hand into the vagina and gently push the presenting part of the fetus back and away from the pulsating cord. This is an acceptable time for you to place your gloved hand into the vagina.

305.
C. This patient's breathing has become inadequate. You must immediately establish an airway and provide positive pressure ventilation.

Seizures and Syncope

306.
B. A seizure is a sudden and temporary alteration caused by the electrical discharge from active foci in the brain.

307.
D. The sequence of events starts with the aura and progresses to the tonic phase lasting 15 to 20 seconds, then to the clonic (tonic-clonic) phase lasting 30 seconds to 5 minutes, and finally to the postictal phase, which lasts from 5 to 30 minutes.

308.
D. Hypoxia is a likely cause of seizure. Other common causes are head injury, stroke, alcohol and drug withdrawal, electrolyte disturbances, hypoglycemia, infection, and high fever in addition to many other causes of seizure.

309.
C. Treatment for an actively seizing patient is supportive. Always protect the patient from harm, maintain the airway, and suction if necessary. Apply oxygen, assist with ventilation if necessary, and transport the patient. Never pry or force anything into the patient's mouth, which can cause further damage.

310.
C. Status epilepticus is a dire medical emergency. These patients need immediate medical intervention.

311.
B. During the tonic phase, the muscles become extremely rigid, and the patient may arch his back.

312.
A. The tonic-clonic phase, also referred to only as the *clonic phase,* usually lasts only 30 seconds to 2 minutes. The muscles alternate between rigidity and relaxation and produce a typical jerky muscle movement.

313.
A. The nasopharyngeal airway can be inserted in an actively seizing patient to provide a means of airway control without harming the patient.

314.
B. Penytoin sodium is the generic name of Dilantin, which is a common medication used to manage seizure disorders.

315.
C. This condition is status epilepticus, a dire medical emergency that requires aggressive airway control and positive pressure ventilation with supplemental oxygen. The patient should be transported rapidly.

316.
C. Syncope usually begins in a standing position. The patient remembers feeling faint or lightheaded. The patient commonly becomes responsive almost immediately after being placed supine. The patient could remember an aura—an abnormal sound, odor, or visual disturbance—that can precede a seizure.

317.
C. The aura is a warning that a generalized tonic-clonic seizure is about to occur. This stage can present as a sound, twitch, or odor; some patients even experience an unusual taste that precedes the seizure. Some patients experience auras; however, many seizure patients do not.

318.

B. The violent and jerky seizure activity caused by alternating relaxation and contraction of muscles is known as the *tonic-clonic* (convulsion) *phase.* An aura can precede a seizure and warn the patient that it is imminent. The tonic phase occurs after the aura and causes the patient to fall to the ground. The patient's muscles become contracted and tense. The hypertonic phase results in severe muscle rigidity. The postictal phase is the recovery phase during which the patient's mental status is altered; however, it progressively improves.

319.

A. The postictal phase is known as the *recovery phase.* During this phase, the patient's mental status can range from complete unresponsiveness to confusion but improves with time. These patients appear exhausted.

320.

C. Syncope usually occurs when the patient is standing or stands up from a sitting position. Syncope is caused by a lack of blood flow to the brain, depriving the brain of oxygen, and rendering the patient unconscious for a brief period. This brief period of unconsciousness is usually corrected after the patient has fallen to a horizontal position.

321.

B. The best position in which to place a patient who has experienced a syncopal episode is supine with the legs elevated. A supine position allows more blood to flow to the brain, increasing cerebral oxygenation. It also allows you to visually inspect the airway and provide oxygen therapy.

322.

B. This emergency situation is most likely a syncopal episode, which usually occurs when the patient is in a standing position and usually resolves after the patient is placed in a horizontal position. The patient often yawns, sways, and then falls to the ground, and the skin is usually moist and pale. The conditon improves when the patient is lying on the ground or floor and the blood flow to the brain is restored.

323.

D. A condition called *Todd's paralysis* can occur during the postictal phase following a tonic-clonic seizure. The weakness or paralysis persists for a brief period of time and resolves itself.

324.

D. A febrile seizure that lasts longer than 15 minutes is considered significant. This patient would require aggressive management.

325.

B. An aura is a warning symptom of a seizure. It can be auditory, visual, or olfactory, or it can be pain sensed in any area of the body. The abdominal pain in this patient is most likely an aura.

5 Trauma

DIRECTIONS Each of the questions or incomplete statements below is followed by suggested answers or completions. Select the **one answer** that is best in each case.

1. Your patient has a laceration to the leg; the wound is bleeding heavily in a steady flow that is dark red. You suspect the patient is bleeding from a:
   A. capillary.
   B. artery.
   C. arteriole.
   D. vein.

2. Which of the following *best* describes arterial bleeding?
   A. dark red blood flows steadily from wounds
   B. bright red blood under high pressure that spurts
   C. oozing flow that usually clots spontaneously
   D. steady flow that is easily controlled with pressure

3. Your adult patient has lost a large amount of blood and is in shock. He is breathing 20 times a minute with good air exchange. You should manage the patient by administering:
   A. oxygen by nasal cannula at 6 lpm.
   B. oxygen by nonrebreather mask at 15 lpm.
   C. positive pressure ventilation.
   D. oxygen by simple mask at 6 lpm.

4. Your patient is bleeding from a laceration to the lateral forearm. The artery or pressure point that should be utilized to control bleeding is the:
   A. ulna.
   B. radial.
   C. femoral.
   D. brachial.

5. A tourniquet to control bleeding should be:
   A. made of a narrow, flat material.
   B. covered with a bandage.

C. used when direct pressure and pressure points fail.
   D. applied directly over a joint tightly enough to eliminate distal pulses.

6. You are treating a patient who is bleeding from the lower leg. Your attempts to control the bleeding with direct pressure are unsuccessful. You should next attempt to control the bleeding by:
   A. utilizing a pressure point.
   B. elevating the extremity.
   C. using a tourniquet.
   D. rapidly apply an air splint.

7. Internal bleeding from blunt trauma:
   A. is usually very obvious to identify.
   B. should be suspected with unexplained shock.
   C. never results in severe blood loss.
   D. can be ruled out if the abdomen is rigid.

8. You and your partner respond to a report of a tree trimmer who fell from a tree. Upon arrival, you find a 34-year-old male lying supine on the ground. The patient presents with signs of severe hypoperfusion. You do not find any signs of external bleeding. Your best immediate treatment for this patient is to:
   A. remain on the scene to determine the exact injury site.
   B. provide immediate transport to the hospital.
   C. transport to the hospital only after advanced life support arrives.
   D. transport to the hospital if the blood pressure decreases.

9. Which of the following are early signs of shock that would alert you that your 20-year-old patient could have internal bleeding from an assault?
   A. decreased blood pressure
   B. deep bradypneic breathing
   C. capillary refill that is 4 seconds
   D. thready pulse at a rate of 110

10. Which signs or symptoms would be unlikely to be found in a hypovolemic patient?
   A. nausea and vomiting
   B. restlessness
   C. warm, flushed skin
   D. marked thirst

11. The outermost layer of the skin that is composed of dead cells and contains the pigment granules is known as the:
   A. epidermis.
   B. endodermis.
   C. dermis.
   D. subcutaneous layer.

12. You and your partner have responded to a patient who was kicked by a horse and sustained a soft tissue injury to the upper thigh. Upon examination of the injured site, you note swelling and pain on palpation. You should first:
   A. control the airway.
   B. administer oxygen.
   C. take body substance isolation precautions.
   D. control the bleeding.

13. A type of soft tissue injury that is caused by scraping, rubbing, or shearing away the epidermis is called a(n):
   A. abrasion.
   B. puncture.

C. avulsion.
D. laceration.

14. You are treating a 34-year-old intoxicated male patient with a stab wound to his anterior chest. What type of dressing should be used to treat the open chest wound?
   A. saline soaked gauze
   B. Vaseline gauze pad
   C. trauma dressing
   D. porous dressing

15. Your patient has an open chest wound. You should secure the occlusive dressing by taping it on:
   A. one side.
   B. two sides.
   C. three sides.
   D. all four sides.

16. You have just arrived on the scene of a reported slashing with a knife. The scene is safe and the police are with the patient. After you expose the patient, you find an open abdominal wound with an evisceration. Emergency care for the evisceration should include:
   A. replacing the abdominal organs.
   B. using a dry absorbent dressing covered in plastic.
   C. keeping the patient's leg flat.
   D. applying a sterile bulky dressing soaked in sterile water.

17. You have responded to an 8-year-old child who has been burned by a grease fire. You notice that large blisters have formed over his arms and chest. You report this as a:
   A. superficial burn.
   B. full thickness burn.
   C. partial thickness burn.
   D. first degree burn.

18. Your patient is suffering intense pain from a scald burn of the epidermis and portions of the dermis. This burn is classified as a:
    A. partial thickness burn.
    B. superficial burn.
    C. full thickness burn.
    D. partial eschar burn.

19. A partial thickness burn involves:
    A. the epidermis only.
    B. the epidermis and dermis.
    C. the dermis and muscle.
    D. the dermis, fat, and muscle.

20. A full thickness burn can appear:
    A. dry, hard, and leathery.
    B. slightly red with blisters.
    C. pink to red.
    D. red with blisters.

21. The classification of a burn that involves the epidermis, dermis, and subcutaneous layers of the skin and often results in an eschar is a:
    A. first degree burn.
    B. full thickness burn.
    C. partial thickness burn.
    D. second degree burn.

22. In managing a full thickness burn, special emphasis should be placed on:
    A. preventing further contamination and injury.
    B. removing clothing that has adhered to the area.
    C. leaving jewelry in the burned areas in place.
    D. calculating the exact body surface area involved.

23. Which of the following is *inappropriate* treatment for the patient with a full thickness burn?
    A. covering the area with a dry sterile dressing
    B. applying a sterile antiseptic burn ointment
    C. administering oxygen by nonrebreather mask
    D. conserving heat loss by covering the patient

24. Which of the following statements is *incorrect* pertaining to the application of pressure dressings?
    A. If blood soaks through, remove and replace dressing.
    B. Air splints can be used to apply pressure on dressing.
    C. Loss of a distal pulse indicates that the dressing is too tight.
    D. The wound should be covered with several bulky dressings.

25. Which of the following impaled objects can be removed in the prehospital setting?
    A. screwdriver embedded in the neck
    B. pitchfork impaled through the foot
    C. pencil impaled through the cheek
    D. knife embedded in the upper leg

26. When managing an electrical burn, the EMT should:
    A. always attempt to remove the patient from the electrical source.
    B. check for a source and ground burn injury.
    C. never attempt CPR unless it is within 4 minutes of contact.
    D. quickly check the pulse, even if the patient is still in contact with the electrical source.

27. Which of the following statements is *incorrect* regarding an electrical injury?
    A. Patients with electrical burns may be treated with the automated external defibrillator (AED) and CPR.
    B. Treatment of a source burn is the same as for other thermal burns.
    C. Injury is usually limited to the area around the source and ground burns.
    D. Patients with burns that appear insignificant are treated as having critical injuries.

28. You are treating a patient who fell from a bicycle and complains of a painful swollen and deformed upper arm. You suspect that the bone injured is the:
    A. scapula.
    B. carpals.
    C. tibia.
    D. humerus.

29. A general rule for splinting is to:
    A. check the pulse, motor function, and sensation before splinting.
    B. check the pulse and sensation before and after splinting.
    C. check the pulse, motor function, and sensation after splinting.
    D. check the pulse, motor function, and sensation before and after splinting.

30. Your patient was struck by a car while riding his bicycle. He complains of pain in his right upper arm and in his back. Which of the following treatments would be *least* desirable for this patient?
    A. elevate the extremity
    B. administer oxygen
    C. apply cold packs
    D. assess motor function

31. Your unit has been dispatched to a local skate park for an injured skater. You find the patient sitting on a bench holding her elbow. Upon examination, you find that the injured area is painful to palpation with noted swelling. When splinting, you should immobilize the:
    A. joint above the elbow joint only.
    B. joint above and below the elbow.
    C. bone above the elbow joint only.
    D. bones above and below the elbow.

32. You are on duty as a standby unit at the local high school soccer game when a player is injured. The patient has an obvious deformity, pain, and swelling to the tibia. The foot is cyanotic and lacks a pulse. You should:
    A. transport the patient immediately without applying a splint and support his leg manually.
    B. apply the splint to his leg in the position found and transport him immediately.
    C. make one attempt to align the extremity by applying gentle manual traction.
    D. make up to three attempts to align the extremity by applying firm traction.

33. Which statement is *false* pertaining to splinting a painful, swollen, or deformed extremity?
    A. Motor, sensory, and distal pulses are assessed both prior to and after splinting.
    B. Joints both above and below should be immobilized when a long bone is injured.
    C. Traction is applied to protruding bones until they retract below the skin.
    D. A pulseless extremity is not aligned by traction if the injury involves the knee.

34. The nervous system that consists of the brain and spinal cord is known as the:
    A. peripheral nervous system.
    B. central nervous system.
    C. voluntary nervous system.
    D. autonomic nervous system.

35. The portion of the skeletal system that protects the brain is the:
    A. vertebrae.
    B. cranium.
    C. calcaneous.
    D. ischium.

36. Which of the following signs and symptoms of spinal injury is rarely seen?
    A. numbness, weakness, or tingling in the arms
    B. pain without movement
    C. obvious deformity of the spine
    D. paralysis of the extremities

37. When performing the primary assessment on a patient with a suspected spine injury, you should open and maintain the airway by:
    A. performing the cervical traction maneuver.
    B. performing the lateral lift maneuver.
    C. performing the head-tilt, chin-lift maneuver.
    D. performing the jaw-thrust maneuver.

38. Placing a patient with a spinal injury on a long spine board is ideally performed by how many rescuers?
    A. two
    B. three
    C. four
    D. five

39. To size a cervical spine immobilization collar, measure the distance from the top of the shoulder to the:
    A. level of the larynx.
    B. bottom of the chin.
    C. level of C-7.
    D. bottom of the earlobe.

40. You arrive on the scene of an automobile crash and find your patient walking around the scene, complaining of neck pain. The correct way to immobilize this patient to minimize movement of the spine is to:
    A. use the standing long board technique.
    B. have the patient sit down on the long board.
    C. use the logrolling technique with a long board.
    D. place the short spinal device on the standing patient.

41. A short spine board is used to immobilize a:
    A. standing patient.
    B. supine patient.
    C. seated patient.
    D. rapid extrication patient.

42. Your patient has been critically injured in a vehicle crash, and he must be transported immediately. You should extricate the patient using the:
    A. short spinal extrication device.
    B. rapid extrication technique.
    C. corset-type immobilization device.
    D. standing long board technique.

43. In which of the following cases should rapid extrication be avoided?
    A. an unsafe scene
    B. a stable patient
    C. a patient blocking access to a critical patient
    D. an unstable patient

44. Which of the following cases would require you to remove a helmet?
    A. The patient has an altered mental status.
    B. The patient complains of head pain.
    C. The patient is in cardiac arrest.
    D. The patient complains of neck pain.

45. The two basic types of helmets are the:
    A. sports and motorcycle.
    B. OSHA and sports.
    C. construction and sports.
    D. construction and motorcycle.

46. When you are dealing with an injured football player with a cervical spine injury, the helmet:
    A. should never be removed under any circumstances.
    B. should be left in place unless a critical need requires removal.
    C. should be removed only by using a special cutting tool.
    D. should always be removed.

Scenario

Questions 47–49 refer to the following scenario:

It is just after 12 A.M. on a Saturday. You have responded to a motor vehicle accident. The patient is in her mid-20s and is walking about the scene. Her car struck a tree, and you note significant damage to its front. The patient appears distraught as you approach. Her right eye is swollen shut and she has a laceration over the left eye. She tells you she had "too much to drink." She is concerned about her car. She complains of neck pain.

47. Given this situation, you should:
    A. have the patient walk to the ambulance and initiate spinal immobilization.
    B. have the patient lie down on the ground and initiate spinal immobilization.
    C. secure the patient's cervical spine and initiate a standing takedown.
    D. have the patient sit down and initiate seated spinal immobilization techniques.

48. During transport to the hospital, the patient begins to complain of a severe headache and dizziness. You should:
    A. repeat your assessment of the level of consciousness.
    B. administer oxygen via nonrebreather mask at 15 lpm.
    C. contact medical direction and ask for assistance.
    D. change your response status from routine to emergency.

49. Her level of consciousness declines, and she now responds to painful stimuli with flexion (decorticate posturing). Your partner also notices a pupillary change from reactive to nonreactive to light. You should:
    A. consider positive pressure ventilation at 20 breaths/minute.
    B. insert an oropharyngeal airway whether a gag reflex exists or not.
    C. pull to the side of the road, reassess the patient, and wait for advanced life support.
    D. continue with your routine response to the hospital and administer oral glucose.

Scenario

Questions 50–52 refer to the following scenario:

You and your partner Bill are responding to a burn emergency. Upon arrival, you find a 52-year-old patient lying supine on the ground next to a gas grill. Bill makes contact with the patient and finds him awake and responsive with an adequate airway. The patient states he was cleaning his grill with gasoline when it exploded and burned him.

50. The patient has sustained burns that encircle both arms; the burns appear dark brown and involve the subcutaneous layer. You classify this burn as a:
    A. superficial thickness burn.
    B. half thickness burn.
    C. partial thickness burn.
    D. full thickness burn.

51. Using the burn severity classification guidelines, you determine that this patient has been critically burned. Which guideline was used to determine this patient's classification?
    A. superficial burn covering 50 percent of body surface area
    B. age of the patient
    C. partial thickness burn covering 20 percent of body surface area
    D. burns encircled both upper extremities

52. You should treat this burn patient by:
    A. covering the burns with dry sterile dressing.
    B. continuing to soak the burns while transporting him.
    C. administering oxygen by nasal cannula at 6 lpm.
    D. removing adhered clothing by pulling gently.

Scenario

Questions 53–55 refer to the following scenario:

You arrive on the scene and find a male patient in his mid-20s who fell from a rocky ledge about 50 feet. Once you gain access to him, you find that he responds to painful stimuli with flexion of his extremities while arching his back. He is bleeding from his mouth, ears, and nose. His respirations are 35/minute and shallow. His radial pulse is present and bounding.

53. Your first immediate action is to:
    A. suction the mouth and apply a nonrebreather mask at 15 lpm.
    B. move the patient up the embankment to the ambulance.
    C. take a set of vital signs.
    D. suction the airway, insert an oropharyngeal airway, and begin bag-valve-mask ventilation.

54. Which of the signs provides the strongest indication that the patient is suffering from a head injury?
    A. the blood coming from the nose, ears, and mouth
    B. a respiratory rate of 35/minute
    C. flexion of the extremities and arching of the back with painful stimuli
    D. strong radial pulses

55. The best treatment you could provide this patient is to:
    A. administer oral glucose to allow the brain cells to function.
    B. maintain a patent airway and continue to provide effective ventilation.
    C. call for advanced life support backup to establish intravenous therapy and fluid resuscitation.
    D. administer oxygen by nonrebreather mask to provide high concentrations of oxygen.

answers & rationales

1.

D. This patient is likely bleeding from a vein. Such bleeding is dark red, has a steady flow, and can be very heavy. Arterial bleeding usually is bright red, very heavy, and spurts with each contraction of the heart. Capillary bleeding is usually slow or oozing and the color is red, but not as bright as it is with arterial bleeding.

2.

B. Arterial bleeding is sometimes difficult to control due its high pressure. Arterial blood is rich with oxygen, which causes it to be bright red. With each contraction of the heart, the artery spurts blood from the wound. Dark red blood with a steady flow describes venous bleeding. Oozing that usually clots spontaneously describes capillary bleeding.

3.

B. This patient is in a hypoperfusion state (shock); breathing is adequate at 20 times/minute with good air exchange. This patient should be administered oxygen by nonrebreather mask at 15 lpm. If the patient's breathing becomes inadequate, you must provide immediate positive pressure ventilation with supplemental oxygen.

4.

D. For bleeding in the upper extremity, the brachial artery or pressure point is utilized. For bleeding from the lower extremity, the femoral pressure point is compressed. Use the heel of one hand for the femoral and the finger tips for the brachial artery.

5.

C. A tourniquet is used only as a last resort to control bleeding. It should be made of a wide, bulky material that will not produce underlying soft tissue injury. The tourniquet should be left uncovered and visible to medical personnel. Avoid placement directly over any joint. The tourniquet should be used after direct pressure and pressure points have failed to control bleeding.

6.

B. If direct pressure fails to control bleeding, you should next try direct pressure with elevation of the extremity. Do not elevate the extremity, however, if a fracture is suspected. A tourniquet is reserved for severe uncontrolled bleeding.

7.

B. Internal bleeding is not always obvious. Suspect internal bleeding if the patient presents with unexplained shock. Patients can lose large amounts of blood internally very rapidly.

8.

B. If you suspect the patient is in shock, you should immediately transport him to the hospital. Do not delay transport to determine the cause of internal bleeding. You should limit the time on the scene, begin transport, and meet advanced life support on the way to the hospital. Patients who are bleeding internally need immediate transport to the hospital where surgical procedures can be performed and blood can be administered. Do not delay transport. Provide oxygen therapy and positive pressure ventilation if necessary.

9.

D. A fast, thready pulse is an early sign of possible internal bleeding and shock (hypoperfusion). Decreased blood pressure is a late sign of shock. Bradypneic breathing indicates a slower than normal breathing rate. The patient in shock usually has a faster than normal breathing rate (tachypnea). A delayed capillary refill in the adult patient is not a reliable sign of hypoperfusion, but it is in a child.

10.

C. The signs and symptoms of hypovolemic shock include restlessness; anxiety; pale, cool, clammy skin; weak pulse; increased pulse rate; increased respirations; decreasing blood pressure (late); dilated pupils; marked thirst; nausea; vomiting; and pallor. The pale and cool skin signs are produced from the constriction of vessels (vasoconstriction) that shunts warm red blood away from the skin. The clammy or sweaty skin is produced from the alpha 1 properties in the epinephrine that is circulating in the body.

11.

A. The outermost protective layer of skin, which is composed of dead cells, is the epidermis. The dermis is the layer below the epidermis and contains nerves, blood vessels, and sebaceous glands. The subcutaneous layer contains the fat and soft tissue and is located below the dermis layer.

12.

C. Because of the obvious hazard of blood and body fluids associated with soft tissue injuries, take body substance isolation precautions prior to patient contact. Be sure to wear gloves, a face mask, and eye protection.

13.

A. An *abrasion* is caused by scraping the outermost layer of the skin or epidermis. It is commonly called a *road rash*. A *puncture* is a penetrating injury that results from a sharp, pointed object entering the soft tissue. An *avulsion* results when a loose flap of skin or soft tissue has been torn loose or pulled completely off. A *laceration* is a break in the skin of varying depth and can be linear (regular) or stellate (irregular).

14.

B. An open wound to the chest should be sealed with an occlusive dressing to prevent air from entering the wound. Occlusive dressings do not permit air to pass through them. These include Vaseline gauze, plastic wrap, and defibrillator pads. The quickest occlusive dressing you can apply is your gloved hand; application immediately seals the wound until a dressing can be applied.

15.

C. Securing the occlusive dressing on three sides allows trapped air within the chest to escape but prevents air outside the chest from entering it. Taping on three sides effectively makes the occlusive dressing a one-way (flapper) valve.

16.

D. The treatment for an open abdominal wound with an evisceration includes covering the organs with a sterile dressing soaked in sterile water or sterile saline. A sterile dressing that is nonadherent is recommended, so avoid using any dressing that can adhere to the organs such as paper, toilet tissue, or paper towels. Place a bulky dressing on top of the sterile water-soaked dressing. This dressing helps to maintain the warmth of the internal organs. Apply an occlusive dressing to cover the entire area and tape it on all four sides. This helps to retain moisture and warmth. Position the patient in a position of comfort, with the hips and knees flexed. Never touch or replace the abdominal organs.

17.

C. Burns are classified as superficial or first-degree burn (red skin), partial thickness or second degree (blisters), and full thickness or third-degree burn (charring).

18.

A. Burns that involve both the epidermis and portions of the dermis are known as *partial thickness* or *second-degree burns*. These burns can be caused by scalding and are painful. Superficial burns, also called *first-degree burns,* involve only the epidermis and are very painful. Full thickness burns involve all three layers of the skin: epidermis, dermis, and subcutaneous layers. The tough and leathery dead soft tissue formed by this burn is called an *eschar.*

19.

B. A partial thickness or a second-degree burn involves the epidermis and dermis. Partial thickness burns cause intense pain from damage to nerve endings.

20.

A. A full thickness burn appears dry, hard, tough, and leathery. It can also appear white and waxy to dark brown or black and charred. The tough and leathery dead soft tissue is called an *eschar.*

21.

B. The full thickness burn involves the epidermis, dermis, and subcutaneous layers of the skin. This type of burn often results in an eschar, or leathery dead soft tissue. The full thickness burn is also known as a *third-degree burn.*

22.

A. Special management of a full thickness burn requires that overall management prevent further contamination and injury to the burn area. Clothing that is adhering to the skin should be left intact because its removal could cause further tissue damage. Remove any jewelry from the hands to prevent restrictive blood flow from swelling that can occur. An *exact* calculation of the body surface area is not required.

23.

B. Never apply any type of ointment or lotion to the burns, it can cause heat retention. Often hospital personnel must then remove the ointment by vigorous cleansing. You should cover the burns with a dry, sterile, particle-free burn dressing. Burn patients often lose too much heat due to damage to their skin, which regulates temperature. Conserve heat loss by covering the patient with blankets. Administer high-flow oxygen by nonrebreather mask if the patient's breathing is adequate and provide positive pressure ventilation.

24.

A. If blood soaks through the dressing, do not remove the dressing because doing so can cause the bleeding to increase. Instead, add additional dressing over the original one and apply pressure.

25.

C. You should never remove an impaled object unless it is impaled through the cheek or in the chest and interferes with chest compressions while performing CPR. Removing impaled objects from areas other than the cheek can lead to further injury or even death. Impaled objects should be stabilized in place using bulky dressings and tape.

26.
B. Never attempt to remove a patient from an electrical source unless you have been trained and are equipped to do so. Check for source and ground burn injury. Never touch a patient who is in contact with an electrical source.

27.
C. An electrical burn can be quite extensive and involve many internal organs such as the heart, spleen, and lungs. If the source burn is on the left hand and the ground burn is on the feet, right hand, hip, knee, and so on, the path crosses the heart and other vital organs. Many electrical burn patients need CPR and defibrillation with the AED. Source and ground burns are treated as thermal burns. Because of the possible involvement of the heart and other vital organs, you should treat all patients with electrical burns as critical patients.

28.
D. The bone of the upper arm is called the humerus.

29.
D. Before and after splinting, check for pulse, motor function, and sensation in the injured extremity. This should be evaluated every 15 minutes after applying the splint to ensure that the splint is not impairing circulation.

30.
A. Do not elevate this patient's extremity because of a possible spinal injury. You should administer oxygen if needed. Application of cold packs can decrease pain and edema (swelling). You should assess the patient's motor and sensory functions and distal pulse before and after applying a splint.

31.
D. When a joint is injured, you should immobilize the bones above and below the affected joint. When a bone is injured, you should immobilize the joints above and below the affected bone.

32.
C. If the extremity is cyanotic and pulseless, you may make one attempt to align it by applying gentle traction to it before splinting. If the pain, resistance, or crepitus increase, you must stop. Do not try to align a wrist, elbow, knee, hip, or shoulder because of major nerves and blood vessels that lie close to these joints.

33.
C. Never intentionally replace a protruding bone into the extremity because this can cause further tissue damage. You should assess the distal pulse and motor and sensory functions before and after applying a splint. To effectively immobilize a long bone, you must immobilize the joint above and below the injured bone. Never try to align an injury that involves the wrist, elbow, knee, hip, or shoulder; doing so can cause more injury.

34.
B. The nervous system that consists of the brain and the spinal cord is the *central nervous system*. The *peripheral nervous system* consists of nerves located outside the brain and spinal cord. The *voluntary nervous system* influences the activity of the voluntary muscles and moves the body. The *autonomic nervous system* influences the activity of involuntary muscles and glands and regulates the heart rate and breathing.

35.
B. The cranium consists of fused bones including the temporal and parietal bones that protect the brain.

36.
C. A rare sign of spinal injury is an obvious deformity of the spine, which is usually found when palpating the spine.

37.
D. Patients with possible spine injuries must be managed carefully. Improper handling can cause further injury or death. When you suspect that a patient could have a spine injury, you must open and maintain the airway using the jaw-thrust maneuver. Cervical traction is not used in the prehospital setting because it can cause further injury including paralysis. Lateral lift or head-tilt maneuvers will compromise the spine and can cause further injury.

38.
C. Ideally, four rescuers perform spinal immobilization and placement on a long spine board. One of them maintains cervical spine stabilization, and the other three perform the logroll maneuver. A fifth rescuer can be used to place the board under the patient.

39.
B. Measure the distance of an imaginary line from the top of the shoulder to the bottom of the chin. Use your fingers to measure the distance.

40.
A. When you encounter a standing patient with a possible spine injury, you must place him onto the board by using the standing long board technique. This technique consists of placing the board behind the patient and lowering him from the standing position. You must maintain control of the patient's head and cervical spine with manual stabilization and the use of a cervical collar. When lowering the patient, support him by placing a rescuer at the side of the board to support him under the arms. All of the other techniques will compromise the spine and possibly cause further injury to the patient.

41.
C. A short spine board or a vest-type device is used to immobilize a patient who is found in a seated position.

42.
B. This patient should be extricated using the rapid extrication technique, which should be used only in the following situations: (1) the scene is not safe (due to fire, explosion, chemical spill, etc.), (2) the patient's condition is so critical and unstable that you need to move and transport him immediately, and (3) the patient blocks your access to a second, more seriously injured patient.

43.
B. Rapid extrication is indicated if the scene is not safe or if the patient's condition is unstable. A stable patient who blocks the access to a second patient who is critically injured may also require rapid extrication. A stable patient does not generally require rapid extrication.

44.
C. If the patient is in cardiac arrest, you must remove the helmet. You should also remove the helmet if it (1) interferes with proper spinal immobilization, (2) does not fit well and allows excessive movement, (3) interferes with your ability to adequately manage the airway or breathing, and (4) interferes with your ability to assess or reassess the airway or breathing.

45.
A. The two basic helmet types are the sports helmet and the motorcycle helmet.

46.
B. The football helmet should be left in place unless there is a life threat that requires its removal. The player's shoulder pads and helmet create a neutral alignment of the spine. Removal of the helmet causes the head to flex.

47.

C. The patient is complaining of cervical spine pain and was involved in an incident with a significant mechanism of injury. Immediately provide cervical spine stabilization and initiate a standing takedown. Do not allow the patient to walk, sit down, or lie down.

48.

A. She could be exhibiting early signs and symptoms of a head injury. It is important to provide a trending of her level of consciousness to determine whether this is, in fact, occurring. Her symptoms could also be a normal response to injury. To determine this, trending of the level of consciousness is required.

49.

A. The level of consciousness is continuing to decline. The EMT should consider providing positive pressure ventilation at a rate of 20 breathsminute because she shows signs of cerebral herniation. These signs include flexion (decorticate) or extension (decerabrate) posturing, pupillary abnormalities such as unequal (one pupil is dilated), or fixed (unreactive) pupils. The patient responds to pain so an oropharyngeal airway is contraindicated. You should change your response to the hospital concerning the emergency as well. The best answer is to consider positive pressure ventilation at a rate of 20 breaths per minute.

50.

D. Burns that involve all layers of the skin including tissue below the subcutaneous layer are classified as *full thickness burns*. They can appear dark brown, black, waxy, dry, hard, leathery, or white. Often the patient with a full thickness burn experiences little pain because the nerve endings are being exposed by the burn.

51.

D. Any burn that encircles a body part (upper extremities, legs, chest, or neck) is classified as a critical burn.

52.

A. You should apply dry sterile dressings after you remove clothing around the area but not that adhered to the skin and initially cool the burn site. Continuing to soak the burn in water could cause hypothermia. Patients who have been burned have lost their temperature-regulating capabilities. This patient's breathing is adequate and does warrant positive pressure ventilation; however, oxygen by nonrebreather mask should be administered.

53.

D. To establish a patent airway and prevent aspiration of the blood, you should immediately suction the airway. Because the patient is not responding appropriately to painful stimuli, you can insert an oropharyngeal airway. Next you should begin positive pressure ventilation because his breathing is shallow.

54.

C. Flexion of the extremities and arching of the back on painful stimulation are indications of an injury to the upper brain stem. This is a form of nonpurposeful posturing, also known as *decorticate posturing.*

55.

B. The best treatment that could be provided to a patient with a head injury is to establish and maintain a patent airway and provide effective ventilation with supplemental oxygen.

6 Infants and Children

DIRECTIONS Each of the questions or incomplete statements below is followed by suggested answers or completions. Select the **one answer** that is best in each case.

1. A child up to 12 months of age is referred to as a(n):
   A. preschooler.
   B. toddler.
   C. neonate.
   D. infant.

2. Which pediatric age group could be classed as the "do-not-like" group? These children generally do not like to be touched, separated from parents, or have clothing removed, and they fear needles. Which group is described?
   A. infant
   B. toddler
   C. preschooler
   D. school age

3. Which pediatric age group uses concrete thinking skills and believes he or she is invincible?
   A. toddler
   B. preschooler
   C. school age
   D. adolescent

4. Which anatomical or physiological difference in the infant and child patient as compared to the adult is correct?
   A. An infant's rib cage is less pliable, resulting in more injury to the ribs.
   B. Infants have a faster metabolic rate that uses oxygen at a faster rate.
   C. Children's heads are proportionally smaller, leading to more head injuries.
   D. A child's skin surface is small compared to body mass, causing hypothermia.

5. Which statement is *incorrect* relating to anatomical differences between the adult and child/infant?
   A. A child's skin surface area is large when compared to body mass.
   B. A child's head is proportionally larger than that of an adult.
   C. An infant has a proportionally larger tongue than that of an adult.
   D. A child has a larger circulating blood volume than that of an adult.

6. An infant or child responds to illness or injury differently than an adult. Which of the following statements best describes a typical *adult's* response to illness or injury?
   A. While crying, the patient says, "It hurts bad."
   B. "Don't touch me!"
   C. "I want to go home!"
   D. "My left arm hurts just below the elbow."

7. The leading medical cause of cardiac arrest in the infant or child patient is:
   A. cardiovascular disease.
   B. drowning or near drowning.
   C. respiratory failure.
   D. seizures.

8. Which is a sign of decompensated or late respiratory failure?
   A. intercostal retractions
   B. nasal flaring
   C. bradypnea
   D. increase in respiratory rate

9. An unresponsive infant or child patient who presents with agonal respirations, limp muscle tone, and a slower than normal heart rate is in:
   A. respiratory arrest.
   B. decompensated respiratory failure.
   C. compensated respiratory failure.
   D. early respiratory failure.

10. Which of the following signs would indicate that an infant or child patient is in decompensated respiratory failure?
    A. neck muscle retraction
    B. "seesaw" respirations
    C. decreased muscle tone
    D. nasal flaring on inspiration

11. An alert, crying child presents with stridor, is pink in color, and is displaying retractions of the intercostal muscles. The mother believes that "something is caught in his throat." The potential problem presented is a _____ that requires you to _____.
    A. partial airway obstruction/place the child in a position of comfort and administer oxygen
    B. partial airway obstruction/administer five back slaps and five chest thrusts
    C. complete airway obstruction/administer five abdominal thrusts
    D. complete airway obstruction/administer five back slaps and five abdominal thrusts

12. Which treatment is indicated for an eight-month infant with a complete airway obstruction?
    A. head-up position while delivering abdominal thrusts
    B. head-up position while delivering chest thrusts and back blows
    C. head-down position while delivering abdominal thrusts
    D. head-down position while delivering back slaps and chest thrust

13. Your partner is preparing to suction an infant; to how many seconds should suctioning be limited?
    A. 5–10
    B. 10–15
    C. 15–20
    D. 20–30

14. Infants and children require a respiratory tidal volume of _____ mL/kg.
    A. 5–10
    B. 10–15
    C. 15–20
    D. 20–25

15. You are treating a severely injured unresponsive child with facial trauma. As you prepare to ventilate the patient with the bag-valve mask, you should *avoid*:
    A. inserting an oropharyngeal airway.
    B. inserting a nasopharyngeal airway.
    C. performing a manual jaw-thrust technique.
    D. maintaining the head in a neutral position.

16. Signs of severe hypoperfusion in children occur _____ because their _____, which helps to maintain the blood pressure.
    A. early/blood vessels constrict
    B. late/blood vessels constrict
    C. late/blood volume increases
    D. early/respiratory rate increases

17. Your patient complains of severe pain and swelling with gross deformity to the proximal right thigh area. The patient presents

with obvious signs of hypoperfusion. Which is *not* a sign of hypoperfusion?

A. pale, cool skin

B. strong peripheral pulse

C. absence of tears when crying

D. decreased urination

18. You and your partner have just assisted in the delivery of a newborn, who should be kept dry and warm following delivery. To what minimum fahrenheit temperature should you heat your ambulance or isollete?

A. 100 degrees

B. 99 degrees

C. 98 degrees

D. 97 degrees

19. The *least* common cause of hypoperfusion in a child is:

A. a cardiac event.

B. diarrhea.

C. dehydration.

D. vomiting.

20. Which is a sign of inadequate perfusion in the infant or child?

A. capillary refill less than 2 seconds

B. warm hands and feet

C. altered mental status

D. normal urinary output

21. Which signs or symptoms could indicate hypoperfusion (shock) in an eight-year-old patient involved in a motor vehicle crash?

A. peripheral pulse of 80/minute

B. bounding peripheral pulse

C. capillary refill of <2 seconds

D. rapid respiratory rate

22. Which is a common cause of seizures in children?

A. epilepsy

B. hypoglycemia

C. overdose

D. fever

23. A seizure in an infant or child that lasts longer than 10 minutes or recurs without a recovery period is called:

A. grand mal activity.

B. mega seizure activity.

C. multiseizure activity.

D. status epilepticus.

24. You are treating a child who was an unrestrained front seat passenger in a motor vehicle crash. Your patient is most likely to have:

A. spine and lower extremity injuries.

B. chest and abdominal injuries.

C. upper extremity and spine injuries.

D. head and neck injuries.

25. The leading cause of death of children from 1 to 14 years of age is:

A. trauma.

B. cardiovascular disease.

C. drowning.

D. asthma.

26. When providing positive pressure ventilation to the injured child, you must take special care to avoid _____, which can be reduced by using _____ during ventilation.

A. gastric distention/cricoid pressure

B. oropharyngeal airway placement/manual airway techniques

C. head movement/head-tilt, chin-lift

D. excessive ventilatory pressures/oropharyngeal airway

27. Which of the following would NOT be an indicator of child abuse?

A. rapidly reporting injuries

B. lack of adult supervision

C. injuries that do not match mechanism

D. a fearful child

28. In most child abuse cases, the child suffers from:
    A. physical abuse.
    B. emotional abuse.
    C. sexual abuse.
    D. physical, emotional, and sexual abuse.

29. Which statement is *incorrect* relating to the care of the potential child abuse patient?
    A. Use subjective information in your patient care report.
    B. Do not make accusatory statements to the parents.
    C. Do not allow the child to be alone with the suspected abuser.
    D. Know the abuse reporting law in your community.

30. What action is frequently required following a call for a traumatic injury to a child or infant?
    A. meeting with local law enforcement personnel
    B. extensive cleaning of the emergency vehicle
    C. debriefing parents and friends
    D. critical incident stress debriefing (CISD) assistance

31. According to the 2010 American Heart Association Guidelines for Cardiopulmonary Resuscitation and Emergency Cardiovascular Care, which of the following describes a *child?*
    A. Less than one year old
    B. One year old to five years old
    C. One year old to eight years old
    D. One year old to the onset of puberty

32. You and your partner have responded to a child in cardiac arrest. Upon arrival on scene, you find a pulseless and apneic five-year-old. When performing chest compressions, you should compress the sternum:
    A. to a depth of one-third the diameter of the chest.
    B. to a depth of one to one and one-half inches.
    C. to a depth of one-half to one inch.
    D. to a depth of two to two and one-half inches.

33. You are treating a six-year-old who was struck by a motor vehicle. The patient presents with an obvious open fracture of the femur with the bone protruding through the skin. You establish manual inline spinal stabilization, and your partner is ventilating the patient. Although the patient has a pulse, you note signs of poor perfusion. When should you begin chest compressions in this patient?
    A. never because the patient has a pulse
    B. if the patient's pulse rate is below 100 beats/minute
    C. if the patient's pulse rate is below 80 beats/minute
    D. if the patient's pulse rate is below 60 beats/minute

34. You arrive on the scene and are met at the street by the parents carrying a limp three-year-old who is not breathing. The mother states that the child stopped breathing approximately 2 minutes ago. You palpate a carotid pulse at 100 beats per minute. You begin ventilation at a rate of:
    A. 6 to 8 breaths/minute.
    B. 8 to 10 breaths/minute.
    C. 12 to 20 breaths/minute.
    D. 22 to 26 breaths/minute.

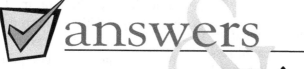
answers & rationales

1.

D. *Neonate* refers to the first four weeks of life, *infant* up to 12 months, *toddler* from one to three years, and a preschooler from three to six years of age.

2.

B. A toddler, a child from one to three years of age, creates an assessment challenge for the emergency responder. Remain calm and try to distract the child with a toy or other object during the assessment.

3.

D. Adolescents (12 to 18 years old) believe that nothing bad can happen to them but are able to use abstract and concrete thinking skills. They may take risks that lead to trauma. If injured, they fear disfigurement and disability.

4.

B. Infants have a faster metabolic rate that uses more oxygen than the adult patient. An infant's rib cage is more pliable, resulting in less rib injury but increased injury to the internal organs.

Children proportionally have larger heads, predisposing them to head injuries. A child's skin surface area is large compared to its mass, which can increase a child's exposure to a cold environment, causing hypothermia.

5.

D. Children have a smaller circulating blood volume than that of adults. Bleeding must be controlled quickly. A seemingly small blood loss in an adult could be life threatening to the infant or child.

6.

D. Children lack the vocabulary and body awareness that adults possess to accurately describe symptoms and assist with care. The adult is able to separate the emotional aspects of illness or injury. The best answer is the most direct answer, "My left arm hurts just below the elbow."

7.

C. The overriding treatment goal for infants and children is to anticipate and recognize respiratory problems. The leading medical cause of cardiac arrest in the infant or child is respiratory failure. Quickly manage and support respiratory compromise in the infant or child patient.

8.

C. Signs of early respiratory distress include intercostal retractions, nasal flaring, increased respiratory rate, supraclavicular and subcostal retractions, neck muscle retractions, audible breathing sounds including stridor, wheezing and grunting, and "see-saw" respirations. The infant or child progresses from early respiratory distress (compensated respiratory failure) to decompensated respiratory failure to respiratory arrest. An infant or child with bradypnea (slow breathing) is a sign of decompensated or late respiratory failure.

9.

A. The signs of respiratory arrest include the signs described in the question as well as weak, absent peripheral pulses and hypotension in patients over three years of age. Patients presenting with these signs require aggressive ventilatory and airway management.

10.

C. In addition to the early signs of respiratory distress (compensated respiratory failure), decreased muscle tone should alert you that your patient is in the advanced stages (decompensated respiratory failure). Neck muscle retraction, "seesaw" respirations, and nasal flaring are all early signs of respiratory distress (compensated respiratory failure).

11.

A. This child patient is presenting with a partial airway obstruction. He is moving air and is pink in color. The treatment for a partial airway obstruction with adequate air movement is to place the patient in a position of comfort, administer oxygen, and encourage the patient to remove the obstruction by coughing.

12.

D. The management of an infant with a complete airway obstruction includes placing the infant in a head-down position during the back slaps and chest thrusts. This position uses gravity to help move the obstruction from the infant airway. Abdominal thrusts are contraindicated in infants.

13.

A. During suctioning of an infant or child's airway, oxygen as well as any debris or secretions is removed. For this reason, limit suctions to no longer than 5–10 seconds.

14.

A. Bag-valve-mask devices that deliver 500 mL to >50 mL should be used to provide positive pressure ventilation to infants and young children. To estimate the volume needed, remember that infants and children require about 5–10 mL per kg of body weight for each ventilation.

15.

B. Avoid the use of a nasopharyngeal airway in adults, infants, and children with possible head trauma and mid-face trauma. Maintaining the head in a neutral position and manual airway control with the jaw-thrust technique is appropriate management.

16.

B. Signs of severe shock, or hypoperfusion, in children occur late because their blood vessels constrict efficiently, which helps to maintain the blood pressure. When the blood pressure does fall, it drops rapidly and quickly. The child or infant can go into cardiac arrest from this rapid drop. When pediatric patients deteriorate because of hypoperfusion, they deteriorate faster and more severely than adults.

17.

B. The peripheral pulse is absent or weak in the child with hypoperfusion. An altered mental status, delayed capillary refill, and a rapid respiratory rate are also present.

18.

C. Heat the ambulance or isollete to a minimum temperature of 98 degrees F (36.5 degrees Celsius). Be sure that the baby's head (not face) is covered to prevent heat loss.

19.

A. Cardiac events in children and infants are uncommon. When they do occur, common causes of hypoperfusion include diarrhea, dehydration, vomiting, trauma, blood loss, infection, and abdominal injuries.

20.

C. Adequate end organ perfusion or tissue perfusion in the infant or child patient is characterized by normal or acceptable findings of capillary refill (2 seconds or less), pulse rate and strength, warm hands and feet, and color of the urinary output, and normal mental status. Alteration of any one of these factors can be an indication of inadequate perfusion.

21.

D. A rapid respiratory rate can indicate hypoperfusion in the child patient. A bounding peripheral pulse does not indicate hypoperfusion; blood is being pumped adequately to the extremities. A capillary refill of <2 seconds is normal.

22.

D. Causes of seizure activity in children and adults are similar with one notable exception, fever. Febrile seizures are common in children but occur rarely in adults.

23.

D. In adults, infants, and children, a seizure that lasts longer than 10 minutes or recurs without a recovery period is called *status epilepticus*. Ensure an airway, be prepared to suction the airway, try to provide positive pressure ventilation, and transport the patient rapidly.

24.

D. Common injury patterns in children who are unrestrained in a vehicle accident include head and neck injuries. This is due to the head size of children and the likely impact of the head with the dashboard.

25.

A. The leading cause of death in children is trauma. This includes vehicle crashes, bicycle accidents, all-terrain vehicle crashes, falls, recreational activities, and pedestrian accidents. The primary killer of children is the automobile.

26.

A. When providing positive pressure ventilation to the injured infant or child, the rescuer must take special care to avoid high ventilatory pressure, which can lead to gastric distention. Gastric distention can be avoided or reduced by using cricoid pressure during ventilation.

27.

A. Rapid reporting of injuries is *not* a general indicator of child abuse. Reports of injuries would be delayed. Additional signs of abuse include multiple abrasions, lacerations, bruises, malnourishment, untreated chronic illness, and injuries on both the front and back or both sides of the child's body.

28.

D. In most child abuse cases, the child suffers from a combination of all of the forms of abuse listed: physical, emotional, and sexual abuse.

29.

A. Document only objective, not subjective, information statements or observations made. Subjective information such as "The patient was abused" must be avoided.

30.

D. CISD for EMTs is frequently required following a call to treat a traumatic injury to an infant or child. Stress and anxiety are common and stem from the EMT lack of experience in treating children, fear of failure, and identification of patients with his own child(ren).

31.

D. According to the 2010 American Heart Association Guidelines for Cardiopulmonary Resuscitation and Emergency Cardiovascular Care, a child is defined as one year old to the onset of puberty (approximately 12 to 14 years old).

32.

A. According to the 2010 American Heart Association Guidelines for Cardiopulmonary Resuscitation and Emergency Cardiovascular Care, a child's chest should be compressed on the lower half of the sternum to a depth of one-third the diameter of the chest.

33.

D. According to the American Heart Association ECC 2005 standards for the health care provider, chest compressions are recommended and should be performed on a child who presents with signs of poor perfusion despite adequate oxygenation and ventilation if the heart rate is less than 60 beats/minute. This trauma patient presents with signs of shock and poor perfusion despite your partner's efforts with ventilations and supplemental oxygen.

34.

C. You should provide ventilation at a rate of 12 to 20 breaths/minute. This rate is approximately one breath every 3 to 5 seconds. Continue to monitor the pulse rate in preparation to begin chest compressions.

7 EMS Operations

DIRECTIONS Each of the questions or incomplete statements below is followed by suggested answers or completions. Select the **one answer** that is best in each case.

1. When you are driving to an emergency scene, most state laws allow:
   A. exceeding the speed limit without regard to the safety for others.
   B. proceeding through a traffic light without regard for the safety of others.
   C. parking anywhere at any time without any restriction.
   D. exceeding the speed limit while respecting the safety of others.

2. You are responding to a medical emergency. Which of the following actions is considered *unsafe* while driving the ambulance?
   A. entering a curve at the outside or high part
   B. accelerating gradually as you leave a curve
   C. driving only as fast as you feel comfortable
   D. braking to the proper speed after entering a curve

3. The use of an escort vehicle is considered dangerous; however, it can be used with extreme caution in which of the following circumstances?
   A. when you are unfamiliar with the way to the hospital
   B. in emergency response to the hospital
   C. when traffic is congested
   D. when responding through an urban area with intersections

4. Which of the following situations is true pertaining to the use of a police escort?
   A. Use escorts only if they allow you to quickly travel through high traffic areas.
   B. Use escorts only at traffic intersections, railroad crossings, and bridges.
   C. Use escorts only if you are unfamiliar with the way to the scene or to the hospital.
   D. Use escorts to reduce the time it takes you to drive through traffic.

5. You are dispatched to an emergency. Which of the following is considered essential patient information in order to respond to the call?
   A. gender
   B. age
   C. name
   D. location

6. You are transporting a critical trauma patient to the hospital. As you approach a railroad crossing, the gates are down and the lights are flashing. You see a long train approaching. You determine that the train is traveling very slowly. You should:
   A. turn on your lights and siren while waiting for the train to pass.
   B. maintain control of the ambulance and cross the tracks quickly.
   C. wait for the train to pass if there is no immediate alternative route.
   D. signal the train to stop and proceed around the warning gates.

7. Which of the following statements is true regarding ambulance-driving techniques?
   A. It is dangerous to brake after entering a curve.
   B. You should accelerate suddenly as you leave a curve.
   C. Stopping distance is shortened when vehicle speed increases.
   D. Brakes in ambulances equipped with antilocking brakes should be pumped.

8. Your patient has vomited on the ambulance floor. Your first action when cleaning the ambulance floor is to:
   A. spread a germicide on top of the vomitus.
   B. sweep the vomitus into a bag with a broom.
   C. clean up visible vomitus with disposable towels.
   D. sterilize the area with a chemical sterilant.

9. Which solution of household bleach to water should be used for intermediate-level disinfecting of surfaces that come into contact with intact skin?
   A. 1:1
   B. 1:10
   C. 1:100
   D. 1:1,000

10. To clean emergency equipment that comes in contact with a patient's intact skin, such as a stethoscope, you should:
    A. immerse it in an EPA-registered sterilant for 6 to 10 hours.
    B. immerse it in an EPA-registered sterilant for 10 to 45 minutes.
    C. use low-level disinfection.
    D. use intermediate-level disinfection.

11. Which of the following best describes the role of the EMT on a scene when a patient is trapped in a motor vehicle?
    A. extrication technician
    B. detanglement worker
    C. patient care provider
    D. scene safety officer

12. You have responded to a motor vehicle crash with the report of injuries and have determined that the vehicle is safe to approach. The most appropriate way to approach the patient trapped in the upright vehicle is:
    A. from the rear of the patient.
    B. directly facing the patient.
    C. from the patient's left side.
    D. from the patient's right side.

13. You have responded to a vehicle crash with injuries and are preparing to extricate the patient using hydraulic tools. Which would be considered inappropriate as you prepare the patient for extrication?
    A. Inform the patient what you are about to do and what to expect.
    B. Instruct the patient to focus on an object directly in front of him.
    C. Have the patient lie across the seat for protection prior to extricating him.
    D. Look the patient directly in the eyes while speaking to him.

14. You have received dispatch information while responding to a call that informs you that the patient will need to be extricated from a vehicle. Your first action should be:
    A. stabilization.
    B. gaining access.
    C. disentanglement.
    D. scene size-up.

15. You have responded to a three-car motor vehicle crash with patients entrapped in the vehicles. The access of choice is usually the:
    A. door.
    B. windshield.
    C. side window.
    D. removed roof.

16. You are on the scene of a two-vehicle crash with heavy damage to the vehicles. After gaining safe access to the patient who is entangled inside one vehicle, you should first:
    A. apply high-flow oxygen.
    B. shake and shout to determine responsiveness.
    C. extricate the patient.
    D. stabilize the cervical spine.

17. The fire officer at the scene of a motor vehicle crash indicates that the patient is entangled in the vehicle and the access appears to be "complex." You recognize that this means that access:
    A. will take longer than 20 minutes.
    B. require the use of tools.
    C. cannot be performed by the EMT.
    D. requires the notification of the police.

18. You have responded to a report of a tractor-trailer that has overturned on the highway. The truck was reported to be hauling hazardous materials. While waiting for the hazardous materials response team to arrive on the scene, you should protect bystanders by:
    A. advising them to shut off electronics.
    B. advising them to remain calm.
    C. directing them to keep downhill.
    D. directing them to keep upwind.

19. You are the first to arrive at the scene of a possible hazardous materials spill at a local factory. Your first action should be to:
    A. ensure that additional equipment and personnel are present.
    B. approach the scene carefully and identify the hazardous material.
    C. protect yourself by donning a hazardous materials protective suit.
    D. secure the scene and prevent exposure to rescuers and bystanders.

20. The area of a hazardous material scene where contamination is actually present and treatment is limited to life-threatening conditions is known as the:
    A. hot zone.
    B. warm zone.
    C. cold zone.
    D. safe zone.

21. The criteria to be considered a multiple casualty incident (MCI) include:
    A. any event that involves mass transit or a large building where people could be located.
    B. any event that places excessive demands on EMS personnel and equipment.
    C. any event that typically involves more than three emergency vehicles.
    D. any event that requires police, fire, and EMS to respond simultaneously.

22. You are the senior EMT and have arrived at the scene of a building collapse with reports of many injured tenants. Your immediate responsibility is to assume the position of:
    A. incident manager.
    B. staging sector manager.
    C. triage sector manager.
    D. supply sector manager.

23. You are the second senior EMT who arrives after the first ambulance on the scene of a school bus overturned on the highway. The first senior EMT initiated the mass casualty incident (MCI) plan. Your immediate role is to assume the position of:
    A. EMS incident manager.
    B. treatment sector officer.
    C. primary triage officer.
    D. staging sector officer.

24. To protect yourself at the scene of a hazardous materials incident, you should position yourself and others:
    A. downhill and downwind.
    B. downhill and upwind.
    C. uphill and downwind.
    D. uphill and upwind.

25. You are on the scene of a multiple casualty incident and have been assigned to the primary triage sector. You open the airway of an unresponsive victim and find that the patient is apneic. You should:
   A. move on to the next patient.
   B. provide rescue breaths for 1 minute.
   C. call for assistance and start CPR.
   D. tag the patient "red" for level one response.

Scenario

Questions 26 and 27 refer to the following scenario:

You and your partner Joshua Adam are cleaning the vehicle as one of your daily chores. The alerting system sounds, "Squad 1, respond to a four-vehicle crash on I-95, mile marker 147, southbound lane." You and Joshua quickly respond. While en route, dispatch advises you of two patients who are critically injured. As you turn onto 20th Street, you notice Squad 7 just ahead of your unit.

26. Your unit is directly behind Squad 7 as you both approach a busy intersection. Which of the following should you do?
   A. Use the same siren mode that Squad 7 is currently using.
   B. Position yourself so motorists can see both units at a glance.
   C. Follow Squad 7 as closely as possible through the intersection.
   D. Follow Squad 7 through the intersection without using your siren.

27. You and Joshua attended to a critically injured trauma patient whom you have transported to the hospital and turned over to the hospital staff with a complete oral and preliminary written report. You and Joshua are standing at the rear of the ambulance, look-

ing with disbelief at the incredible mess you both created while attending to the trauma patient. After you both have picked up all the loose trash and cleaned all of the blood from the inside of the ambulance, Joshua states that he will clean the laryngoscope blades. Which of the following best describes the correct procedure for cleaning them?
   A. Immerse them in an EPA-registered sterilant for 10 to 45 minutes.
   B. Immerse them in an EPA-registered sterilant for 6 to 10 hours.
   C. Wipe them carefully with a 1:10 solution of bleach and water.
   D. Wipe them carefully with a 1:100 solution of bleach and water.

Scenario

Questions 28–30 refer to the following scenario:

You and your partner Russ are reviewing your department's protocol when the alerting system sounds: "Squad 1, respond to an automobile crash with injuries at 1729 17th Avenue." You both quickly move to the ambulance. While you are en route to the accident scene, dispatch advises you that a bystander stated that nine persons are injured, some of whom could be in critical condition. You advise dispatch to activate the multiple casualty incident (MCI) plan.

28. What criterion did you use to determine that the MCI plan needs to be implemented?
   A. This event will likely take longer than 2 hours to complete.
   B. This event and location will limit the number of rescuers on the scene.
   C. This event will require an emergency response from EMS, fire, and police.
   D. This event will likely place excessive demand on personnel and equipment.

29. Your unit is the first to arrive on the crash scene and you are the most senior EMT. Your initial role is as primary:

    A. triage manager.
    B. incident manager.
    C. treatment manager.
    D. staging manager.

30. Your partner Russ is assigned to the triage sector. *Triage* is best described as a system:

    A. ensuring that ambulances are accessible and transportation occurs with direction of EMS incident manager.
    B. responsible for distributing the medical material and equipment necessary to render care.
    C. that monitors, inventories, and directs available emergency ambulances to the treatment sector.
    D. used to sort patients to determine the order in which they will receive care and transport.

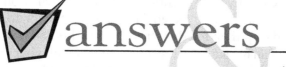

answers
& rationales

1.

D. When operating an ambulance, you must always respect the safety of others, called *due regard for the safety of others.* This due regard must followed when you travel through a traffic light, park, or exceed the speed limit.

2.

D. Braking to the proper speed after entering a curve is considered unsafe. You should decelerate to a safe speed prior to entering the curve.

3.

A. The only acceptable use of an escort vehicle is when the driver of the ambulance is unfamiliar with the way to the hospital. When using an escort, exercise extreme caution.

4.

C. You should use a police escort only if you are uncertain of how to reach the scene or the hospital.

5.

D. The location of the patient is considered essential information needed to respond to a call. Neither the gender nor the age is essential information; however, it is often included as additional information. The name of the patient should not be given over the radio; doing so can be considered a breech of patient confidentiality.

6.

C. *Never* proceed through a crossing gate at a railroad crossing! Simply be calm and monitor your patient. If there is no immediate alternative route, wait for the train to pass. Turning on your lights and siren while waiting for the train to pass is likely to upset the patient and others.

7.

A. After entering a curve, it is dangerous to apply the brakes. Anticipate the curve and apply the brakes before entering the curve; accelerate gradually and carefully as you leave it. Stopping distances increase as the speed of the vehicle increases. Ambulances equipped with antilocking brakes should not be pumped; apply the brakes firmly and steadily.

8.

C. When cleaning any body fluid or substance that has spilled, you should first remember to wear gloves, a mask, and eyewear. Clean it by using disposable towels to pick up the majority of the spill. After you have picked up the spill and disposed of it properly, you need to clean the surface with a germicide or mixture of bleach and water. Never try to pick up a spill with a broom, which only creates a larger spill and could cause additional contamination.

9.

B. A ratio of 1:10, or 1 part household bleach to 10 parts water, is the correct mixture to use for an intermediate-level disinfection. A 1:1 mixture is too strong; a 1:100 ratio is too weak for an intermediate-level disinfection but is used for a low-level disinfection such as routine cleaning of the ambulance. A 1:1,000 mixture is too weak.

10.

D. When cleaning equipment that comes in contact with the patient's intact skin, use an intermediate-level disinfectant (1:10 ratio of bleach to water). A ratio of 1:100 is used for routine housekeeping on surfaces such as floors. Equipment that comes in contact with a patient's mucous membranes should be soaked for 10 to 45 minutes in an EPA-registered sterilant. Immersion in an EPA-registered sterilant for 6 to 10 hours is used on equipment that is used invasively, primarily in the hospital.

11.

C. Your primary role as an EMT at a crash scene is as a patient care provider. Although you will work closely with the detanglement team and help to ensure minimal risk to the patient's condition, you will provide emergency care to the patient.

12.

B. When approaching a patient inside a vehicle, you should approach directly facing the patient. Approaching the patient from his front helps to keep the patient's attention forward, thus keeping him from turning his head. When you have made direct eye contact with your patient, instruct him not to move his head. Approaching from the right, left, or behind can cause the patient to move his head, possibly causing further injury to the patient.

13.

C. Having the patient lie across the seat could cause further injury. You must maintain in-line spinal stabilization during extrication. It is important to explain to your patient what to expect; this will lessen his apprehension during the extrication process. Having the patient focus on an object directly in front of him helps to keep his head and spine in line and still. When speaking to your patient, look him directly in the eyes; this helps keep the patient from moving his head unnecessarily.

14.

D. You first must size up the scene; this helps you to organize your resources and prepare for the extrication. A good scene size-up can help reduce injury to the rescuers and the patient.

15.

A. The door is usually the best access when extricating a patient from a motor vehicle because of its large opening. In addition, it normally is fairly easy to open. The windshield can be difficult through which to gain access. The side window is usually too small and could cause the spine to be manipulated. The removal of the roof opens the vehicle considerably and can make extrication much easier but usually requires special training and equipment and can be costly to the vehicle owner.

16.

D. After gaining safe access to your patient, you will stabilize the cervical spine with manual in-line stabilization. Provide the same care as you would for other trauma patients. Apply high-flow oxygen after securing the cervical spine manually. Shaking and shouting to establish responsiveness can cause the patient to move, injuring an unsecured cervical spine.

17.

B. Complex access requires the use of tools or specialized equipment. Access that does not require tools or specialized equipment is known as "simple access."

18.

D. While waiting for help to arrive on a hazardous materials incident, you should protect bystanders (and yourself) by having them keep upwind (or uphill and away from the scene). Turning off electronics will not protect you from hazardous materials.

19.

D. As the first responding EMT on the scene of a hazardous material incident, you should first secure the scene, which will limit the exposure to other rescuers and bystanders.

20.

A. The *hot zone* is where contamination is actually present. Trained personnel wearing protective equipment provide treatment in this area. Treatment is limited to life-threatening conditions. The *warm zone* is the area outside the hot zone where patients and personnel must remain until they are fully decontaminated. The *cold* or *safe zone* is outside the warm zone and is where personnel can remove protective clothing; all life-threatening conditions should have been attended to before the patient reaches this zone.

21.

B. An MCI is typically defined as any event that places excessive demands on EMS personnel and equipment. This criterion is specific to your individual system. Often an incident involving mass transit or a large building can turn into a MCI; however, the incident must meet the stated criterion. The response of three emergency vehicles could tax a rural system but not another system. Often many events routinely require police, fire, and EMS to respond simultaneously.

22.

A. The senior EMT who arrives at the scene of a disaster first assumes the EMS incident manager position until relieved by the predesignated officer. The predesignated officer who relieves the EMT may reassign him as a sector officer.

23.

C. Your immediate role as the second senior EMT on an MCI is as the primary triage officer. Remain at this post until the EMS incident commander relieves you.

24.

D. To protect yourself and others from possible exposure of a hazardous materials incident, you should position yourself and others uphill and upwind. Positioning in this manner limits exposure because many chemicals are carried with the wind, liquids flow downhill, and some gasses are heavier than air.

25.

A. It can be difficult to do, but you must move on to the next patient if you find that there is no breathing or no pulse. Providing emergency care to this patient would take too many of your much-needed resources and could cause additional loss of life.

26.

B. You should position your vehicle at a safe distance behind Squad 7 but close enough so that motorists can see both units at a glance. Do not follow too closely; reaction time decreases, and motorists could think that there is only one emergency vehicle and proceed, possibly striking your vehicle. Always use all of your lights and siren when you approach and proceed through an intersection. When following another emergency vehicle, use a different siren mode than the other vehicle uses.

27.

A. Equipment that comes in contact with mucous membranes such as laryngoscope blades should be cleaned by soaking it in an EPA-registered sterilant for 10 to 45 minutes. Hospitals usually soak their invasive equipment in an EPA-registered sterilant for 6 to 10 hours. Simply wiping the blades with a 1:100 or 1:10 bleach and water solution will not disinfect them adequately.

28.

D. This event will likely place an excessive demand on personnel and equipment resources. It is far better to activate the MCI plan and have too many rescuers and equipment en route to the scene than too few.

29.

B. If you are the most senior EMT to arrive on the scene of a multiple casualty incident, your initial role is that of the EMS incident manager until the predesignated officer, if there is one, relieves you.

30.

D. *Triage* is a system that sorts patients to determine the order in which they will receive care and transportation to the hospital. Triage usually divides patients into groups who are high priority, second priority, and lowest priority.

8 Advanced Airway Management

DIRECTIONS Each of the questions or incomplete statements below is followed by suggested answers or completions. Select the **one answer** that is best in each case.

1. The depression that is located between the base of the tongue and the epiglottis is known as the:
   A. vallecula.
   B. glottic opening.
   C. vocal cords.
   D. larynx.

2. The space between the true vocal cords where the endotracheal tube is placed is known as the:
   A. glottic opening.
   B. vallecula.
   C. larynx.
   D. epiglottis.

3. The narrowest portion of the infant's airway is at the level of the:
   A. true vocal cords.
   B. laryngopharynx.
   C. cuneiform cartilage.
   D. cricoid cartilage.

4. Because the head is proportionately larger in children than in adults, padding should *not* be placed under the head of a child younger than:
   A. 9 years of age.
   B. 11 years of age.
   C. 13 years of age.
   D. 15 years of age.

5. Which statement is true regarding airway compromise in children?
   A. Because the tongue is larger in a child than in an adult, it is the most common cause of airway obstruction.
   B. Most airway obstructions in the child patient are caused by a foreign body lodged in the carina.
   C. Because a child's head is smaller than that of an adult, it is less likely to flex the neck forward, thus compromising the airway.
   D. The trachea is firmer and less flexible, which likely will cause an airway compromise.

6. You have responded to a patient who has fallen from a roof approximately 30 feet to the concrete parking lot. The patient is responding to verbal stimuli. Which of the following will help maintain an open airway?
   A. oropharyngeal airway
   B. head-tilt, chin-lift
   C. head-tilt, extension technique
   D. nasopharyngeal airway

7. Insertion of a nasogastric tube is indicated in which of the following?
   A. A four-year-old child who was involved in a bicycle accident and sustained significant facial trauma
   B. A two-year-old child for whom you cannot provide effective ventilation due to gastric distention
   C. A one-year-old child who complains of a painful throat and has a seal-like bark when he coughs
   D. A three-year-old child who may have ingested a caustic chemical substance such as drain cleaner

8. The procedure that applies pressure on the cricoid cartilage, closing off the esophagus and reducing the chance of aspiration, is called:
   A. Trendelenburg position.
   B. McIntosh pressure.
   C. Buck's extension.
   D. Sellick's maneuver.

9. In which of the following patients would orotracheal intubation be contraindicated?
   A. 54-year-old patient without a gag reflex who cannot protect his or her own airway
   B. 34-year-old unresponsive patient who will not tolerate an oropharyngeal airway
   C. 18-year-old patient with mouth trauma for whom you are unable to get a good seal with the mask
   D. 73-year-old cardiac arrest patient with a history of cardiomegaly

10. Which laryngoscope blade is preferred for intubating infants and children?
    A. curved
    B. McIntosh
    C. convex
    D. Miller

11. Which laryngoscope blade lifts the epiglottis indirectly by pressing on the glossoepiglottic ligament?
    A. Miller
    B. Wisconsin
    C. Flagg
    D. McIntosh

12. The straight laryngoscope blade exposes the vocal cords and the glottic opening by:
    A. indirectly lifting the epiglottis.
    B. fitting into the vallecula.
    C. directly lifting the epiglottis.
    D. pressing the glossoepiglottic ligament.

13. Which is incorrect regarding a malleable stylet used in endotracheal intubation?
    A. The stylet provides stiffness to alter the shape of the tube.
    B. The stylet should be lubricated with a water-soluble lubricant.
    C. The stylet should extend past the Murphy eye 1 to 2 cm.
    D. The stylet must be recessed one-half inch from the distal end.

14. In the emergency setting, which size of endotracheal tube usually fits both the adult male and female?
    A. 6.5 mm i.d.
    B. 7.0 mm i.d.
    C. 7.5 mm i.d.
    D. 8.0 mm i.d.

15. You have responded to a two-year-old who is in cardiac arrest. Which formula is used to estimate the correct size of the endotracheal tube for this child?
    A. Tube size = (Age in months + 16) ÷ 2
    B. Tube size = (4 ÷ Age in years) + 4
    C. Tube size = (Age in months × 4) ÷ 16
    D. Tube size = (16 + Age in years) ÷ 4

16. Which of the following complications are you least likely to encounter while intubating the adult patient?
    A. tachycardia
    B. arrhythmia
    C. hypotension
    D. hypoxia

17. An alternative method for estimating the size of the endotracheal tube needed for a child is to choose:
    A. a tube with the same outside diameter as the patient's little finger.
    B. a tube with an inside diameter the same as the patient's fingernail.
    C. by measuring from the tip of the patient's nose to the angle of the lower jaw.
    D. a tube that is slightly larger than the patient's glottic opening.

18. You are preparing to intubate your adult patient. You should ventilate the patient at a rate of:

    A. 10 to 12 breaths/minute for 1 to 2 minutes.

    B. 18 to 20 breaths/minute for 2 to 4 minutes.

    C. 20 to 24 breaths/minute for 1 to 2 minutes.

    D. 24 to 28 breaths/minute for 1 to 3 minutes.

19. When preparing to intubate a nontraumatic patient, which of the following is an *inappropriate* technique to maximize visualization of the vocal cords?

    A. placing a folded towel under the patient's shoulder blades

    B. positioning the patient's head in a sniffing position

    C. positioning the head backward while lifting the chin forward

    D. placing the patient's head so that it hangs over the edge of the bed

20. Of the following, the correct sequence for inserting the laryngoscope is to:

    A. hold the laryngoscope in the left hand, insert it into the right corner of the mouth, and sweep the tongue to the left.

    B. hold the laryngoscope in the right hand, insert it into the right corner of the mouth, and sweep the tongue to the left.

    C. hold the laryngoscope in the left hand, insert it into the left corner of the mouth, and sweep the tongue to the left.

    D. hold the laryngoscope in the left hand, insert it into the left corner of the mouth, and sweep the tongue to the right.

21. An indication that you have successfully intubated your patient with an endotracheal tube is when:

    A. the distal cuff inflates and secures the tube in place.

    B. you are able to visualize the tube pass through the glottic opening.

    C. you are able to place the tube through the oval esophageal opening.

    D. you hear air rush into the patient's mouth and nose.

22. After you witness the endotracheal tube pass through the vocal cords, you hear lung sounds to only the right chest. You should:

    A. deflate the cuff and extubate the patient; then try again.

    B. deflate the cuff and withdraw the tube slightly; then re-inflate.

    C. gently advance the tube forward and add air to the cuff.

    D. ask the patient whether his right lung has been surgically removed.

23. Your partner has intubated a patient. After assessing for proper placement, you are unsure whether the endotracheal tube has been properly placed. You should:

    A. leave the tube in place and reassess.

    B. deflate the cuff and pull back gently.

    C. perform a rapid medical assessment.

    D. immediately remove the tube.

24. You and your partner are attempting to intubate an infant who has poor ventilation following a seizure. As you proceed with the intubation attempt, you notice that his heart rate has fallen below 80 beats/minute. You should:

    A. continue the intubation attempt and start CPR immediately.

    B. stop the intubation attempt and hyperoxygenate with a bag-valve-mask (BVM) device.

    C. continue the intubation attempt and insert an oropharyngeal airway.

    D. stop the intubation attempt and perform a finger sweep.

25. The best indicator of proper endotracheal tube placement in infants and children is:
   A. auscultating bilateral breath sounds anteriorly.
   B. watching the diaphragm move by observing the abdomen.
   C. observing changes in the pulse oximeter device.
   D. observing the symmetrical rise and fall of the chest.

26. Insertion of an oropharyngeal airway (OPA) after intubating a child is recommended because:
   A. the OPA acts as a bite block.
   B. the OPA keeps the tongue forward.
   C. the OPA helps to secure the tube.
   D. the OPA keeps the airway open.

27. You have successfully intubated your infant patient when you notice inadequate lung expansion. Which of the following can cause the inadequate lung expansion?
   A. The tube is too small for this patient.
   B. The tube has become blocked by secretions.
   C. There is a leak in the bag-valve-mask.
   D. All of the above can cause it.

28. Confirming correct endotracheal tube placement is accomplished by:
   A. auscultating over the epigastrium.
   B. watching for chest rise and fall.
   C. auscultating breath sounds.
   D. All of the above can confirm it.

29. While treating a cardiac arrest patient, you suspect that your partner has intubated the esophagus. You should:
   A. extubate and hyperoxygenate with a bag-valve-mask (BVM) device.
   B. extubate and reattempt to intubate the patient.
   C. leave the tube in place and intubate around it.
   D. leave the tube in place and hyperoxygenate with a device.

30. After you have successfully intubated your child patient, which of the following helps limit the possibility of a dislodged tube?
   A. inflating the cuff with 10 cc of air
   B. inserting an oropharyngeal (OPA) airway
   C. immobilizing the patient's head
   D. deactivating the pop-off valve

Scenario

Questions 31–34 refer to the following scenario:

You and your partner Mim are taking a well-deserved break at the station when the station alerting system sounds: "Squad 1, respond to a respiratory call at 455 Nell Avenue." You put down your coffee and pick up your run report computer and walk briskly to the ambulance. Upon arriving at the scene and ensuring that it is safe, you enter the patient's house. The husband leads you to a back bedroom where you find the patient, a 68-year-old female, lying on the floor unresponsive to any stimulus and breathing 6 times a minute. Mim, being the more senior and experienced EMT, decides not to insert an airway adjunct and hyperoxygenate the patient with the bag-valve-mask (BVM) device but to intubate this patient with an endotracheal tube.

31. Why did Mim decide to intubate this patient rather than to ventilate with the BVM and airway adjunct?
   A. The patient is unresponsive to any type of stimulus.
   B. The bag-valve-mask is contraindicated in this patient.
   C. This patient will not tolerate an airway adjunct.
   D. The patient's age dictates the endotracheal tube is needed.

32. Mim chooses to use the McIntosh (curved) blade to intubate the patient. Which best describes the correct sequence and technique for using the McIntosh blade?
    A. Enter the mouth on the left side, sweep the tongue to the right, and lift the epiglottis directly.
    B. Enter the mouth on the right side, sweep the tongue to the left, and lift the epiglottis directly.
    C. Enter the mouth on the right side, sweep the tongue to the left, and lift the epiglottis indirectly by placing the tip of the laryngoscope blade into the vallecula.
    D. Enter the mouth on the left side, sweep the tongue to the right, and lift the tongue indirectly.

33. Mim observes the tube pass through the vocal cords and glottic opening and holds the tube securely in place and inflates the distal cuff by injecting air. How much air should be injected?

A. 1 to 3 cc
B. 5 to 10 cc
C. 15 to 20 cc
D. 20 to 30 cc

34. Immediately after passing the endotracheal tube, you should first assess for tube placement by:
    A. auscultating over the 2nd intercostal space on the midclavicular line.
    B. auscultating over the epigastrium.
    C. watching for an increase on the pulse oximeter.
    D. feeling for resistance when squeezing the bag-valve device.

35. The size of the average endotracheal tube used in the adult male patient is _____ mm.
    A. 6.0
    B. 7.0
    C. 7.5
    D. 8.0

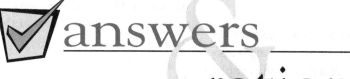

answers & rationales

1.

A. The depressed space between the epiglottis and the base of the tongue is the vallecula. The McIntosh (curved) laryngoscope blade fits into the vallecula to indirectly lift the epiglottis during endotracheal intubation.

2.

A. The area between the true vocal cords is known as the *glottic opening.* You must actually see the endotracheal tube pass through the glottic opening to be certain that the tube is being placed correctly.

3.

D. The narrowest portion of the airway in an infant and a child is the cricoid cartilage. It is important to remember this because the endotracheal tube can pass easily through the vocal cords but be too large to pass the cricoid ring.

4.

A. The head of a child under the age of 9 years is proportionately larger. Placing a pad under the head could occlude the airway by flexing the head and neck forward.

5.

A. The tongue is larger in the child than the adult and is the most common cause of airway obstruction. Often, a foreign body lodges at the level of the cricoid cartilage because this is the narrowest portion of the pediatric airway anatomy. Proportionately, the child's head is larger than that of an adult and can easily flex the neck forward, compromising the airway. Because a child's trachea is not as firm and is more flexible than that of the adult, this can cause an airway compromise.

6.

D. The nasopharyngeal airway helps to maintain an adequate airway in a trauma patient. The oropharyngeal airway is contraindicated in a responsive patient. Movement of the patient's head is contraindicated in the trauma patient.

7.

B. If you are unable to effectively ventilate your pediatric patient because of gastric distention, you should relieve the pressure by inserting a nasogastric tube. Its use is contraindicated in patients with facial trauma.

8.
D. Sellick's maneuver is a procedure that applies pressure to the cricoid cartilage by pressing backward on the Adam's apple, closing off the esophagus, thus reducing the chance of aspiration. The Trendelenburg position is also known as the *shock position;* it elevates the feet slightly above the head while the patient is in the supine position. Buck's extension refers to Gurdon Buck, an early American surgeon who invented a device made of a weight and a pulley for applying extension to a limb.

9.
B. A patient who will not tolerate an oropharyngeal airway is not likely to accept orotracheal intubation. You should intubate a patient without a gag reflex who cannot protect his own airway, who has mouth trauma and for whom you are unable to maintain an adequate mask seal, and who is in cardiac arrest. *Cardiomegaly* describes the patient's history of hypertrophy (increased size) of the heart.

10.
D. The Miller (straight) blade is preferred when intubating infants and children. It provides better displacement of the tongue and allows for better visualization of the glottic opening. The Macintosh blade is curved or convex.

11.
D. The curved or McIntosh laryngoscope blade lifts the epiglottis indirectly. The tip of the McIntosh blade is inserted into the vallecula where it presses the glossoepiglottic ligament, lifting the epiglottis. The other blades are straight and lift the epiglottis directly.

12.
C. The straight blade (Miller, Wisconsin, or Flagg) lifts the epiglottis directly by placing the tip under the epiglottis and lifting. The other distracters describe the curved or McIntosh blade.

13.
C. The Murphy eye is located at the distal end of the tube, and the stylet should not extend past this area. Extending the stylet beyond the Murphy eye can injure the patient.

14.
C. The 7.5 mm i.d. endotracheal tube usually fits both the adult male and female in the emergency setting.

15.
D. The following is the correct formula to estimate the endotracheal tube size for a child over the age of one year: Tube size = (16 + Age in years) ÷ 4. Thus, the correct size for a four-year-old child is 5 (16 + 4 = 20; 20 ÷ by 4 = 5). The patient should receive a 5.0 mm i.d. endotracheal tube.

16.
C. Hypotension is rarely seen when intubating the adult patient, but tachycardia, arrhythmia, and hypoxia are common complications.

17.
A. To estimate the correct endotracheal tube size for a child, select a tube with the same outside diameter as the child's little finger. Never choose a tube larger than the glottic opening.

18.
A. The adult patient needing to be intubated should be hyperoxygenated at a rate of 10 to 12 breaths/minute for 1 to 2 minutes.

19.
D. Never place the patient's head in a position that does not allow for support; this could cause serious injury. Each of the others is an appropriate technique for the nontraumatic patient.

20.
A. The correct sequence for inserting the laryngoscope, which will help to maximize sight of the vocal cords and the glottic opening, is to hold the scope in the left hand, insert it into the right corner of the mouth, and sweep the tongue to the left.

21.
B. When you visualize the endotracheal tube pass directly through the glottic opening, you can be sure that the tube has been correctly placed. Beware, however; just because the tube has been placed correctly does not mean that it cannot become dislodged and then intubate the esophagus. The purpose of the distal cuff is to seal the airway, not to secure the tube in place. Placing the tube and leaving it in the esophagus is a grave mistake and will cause the patient to die. If the patient is properly intubated and the cuff inflated, you should not hear air escaping.

22.
B. After the tube has passed through the glottic opening and lung sounds are heard on only the right side of the chest, the tube is likely in the right mainstem bronchus. You should carefully deflate the cuff and gently withdraw the tube 1 to 2 cm. Next, re-inflate the cuff and recheck the lung sounds. A lobectomy (surgical removal of lung) on the right side of the chest causes the absence of lung sounds.

23.
D. If at any time you are unsure whether the endotracheal tube has been properly placed, you should immediately remove it. It is far better to remove the tube and ventilate with a bag-valve-mask device than to leave the tube in place, which will cause the death of the patient and could subject you to litigation.

24.
B. If the heart rate falls below 80 beats/minute in the infant, this is an ominous sign of hypoxia. You should immediately stop the intubation attempt and hyperoxygenate the patient with the BVM with supplemental oxygen.

25.
D. The best indicator of proper endotracheal tube placement in the infant or child patient is watching the symmetrical (both sides) rise and fall of the chest. Lung sounds can be deceiving in the infant and child. Pulse oximeter may not have an immediate effect in these patients. Watching the abdomen move is not a good indication of proper tube placement.

26.
A. The OPA acts as a bite block and prevents the patient from biting the soft tube and obstructing the airflow. There is no reason to keep the tongue forward; the endotracheal tube is an airway that directly isolates the trachea. The OPA does not secure the tube. There is no need to keep the airway open because the endotracheal tube has been directly inserted into the traceha.

27.
D. After you see the endotracheal tube pass directly through the vocal cords and you are sure that it has been properly placed, you notice poor tidal volume. You should assess the patient and equipment: Is the tube too small for this patient?

Does the bag-valve-mask device have a leak or a pop-off valve? Is the EMT delivering enough tidal volume? Has the tube become blocked?

28.
D. Each of these is used to confirm the correct placement of the endotracheal tube.

29.
A. If you suspect that the endotracheal tube has been placed into the esophagus, you must immediately extubate (remove) the tube and hyperoxygenate the patient. You must not attempt to re-intubate the patient until he has been hyperoxygenated. The placement of the first tube in the esophagus does not ensure that the next will be placed into the trachea. The esophagus is elastic and can easily accommodate two tubes. Intubating the esophagus and leaving the tube in place are lethal mistakes. Trying to ventilate a patient with a BVM around a tube will prevent a good mask seal.

30.
C. Immobilizing the child's or infant's head will reduce movement, which can help limit the possibility of a dislodged tube. Inflating the cuff only seals the tube but does not help to secure it. Inserting an OPA can act as a bite block but will not help secure the tube. When you are ventilating a patient, the pop-off valve should always be deactivated.

31.
A. Mim is correct in choosing to intubate this patient because she does not respond to any stimulus. By intubating this patient, you establish a secure airway that the patient cannot protect on her own. Use of the BVM and an airway adjunct, could cause the patient to vomit and aspirate into the lungs. The BVM and airway adjunct are not contraindicated in this type of patient; however, the best choice is orotracheal intubation if your medical direction permits it.

32.
C. The correct technique for using the curved McIntosh blade to intubate a patient is to enter the mouth from the right side, sweep the tongue to the left, and lift the epiglottis indirectly by inserting the tip of the blade into the vallecula.

33.
B. The distal cuff should be inflated with 5 to 10 cc of air. Overfilling the cuff could cause injury to the trachea. Underfilling the cuff could cause air to escape around the tube, resulting in an inadequate air exchange. Moreover, an underfilled cuff might not prevent secretions from entering the airway.

34.
B. Immediately after passing the endotracheal tube, you should listen over the epigastrium for sounds in the stomach, which would indicate that the tube is in the esophagus. If so, you would immediately remove the tube. After the epigastrium, you would auscultate the chest at the 2nd intercostal space midclavicular and then 4th intercostal space midaxillary. At the same time, you would inspect the chest for adequate rise and fall.

35.
D. The size of the average endotracheal tube used in the adult male patient is 8.0 mm. An adult female typically takes a 7.5 mm size tube.

Comprehensive Exam

1. An example of an unsafe on-the-scene activity is:
   A. wearing reflective clothing at night.
   B. using latex gloves.
   C. wearing protective clothing.
   D. entering a crime scene quickly.

2. Which of the following is a behavioral response to stress?
   A. depression
   B. overeating
   C. defensiveness
   D. mood swings

3. The single most important way to prevent the spread of infection is by:
   A. wearing latex gloves.
   B. wearing a disposable facemask.
   C. using antiseptic wipes.
   D. washing your hands vigorously.

4. While en route to a residence that is the scene of a stabbing, a bystander informs dispatch that the patient is bleeding heavily. You should:
   A. make patient contact and immediately begin your treatment.
   B. gain access to the residence and speak to the patient from a distance.
   C. wait for police to secure the scene before entering it.
   D. position your vehicle at the side of the residence and wait for police to arrive.

5. Which of the following would require special reporting?
   A. abuse
   B. fall
   C. asthmatic attack
   D. cardiac arrest

6. What anatomical term means "on both sides"?
   A. unilateral
   B. lateral
   C. bilateral
   D. proximal

7. What type of joint is the shoulder?
   A. gliding
   B. pivot
   C. ball and socket
   D. hinged

8. Which of the following patients is breathing adequately?
   A. 6-month-old breathing with abdominal muscles at 20 times a minute
   B. 42-year-old breathing irregularly from sighs at 20 times a minute
   C. 8-year-old breathing with accessory muscles at 30 times a minute
   D. 60-year-old breathing with unequal chest expansion at 22 times a minute

9. You are treating an eight-year-old patient who was kicked in the head by a horse. You should open the airway by using:
   A. a jaw-thrust maneuver.
   B. a head-tilt, chin-lift maneuver.
   C. head-tilt, neck-lift maneuver.
   D. padding under the shoulders to flex the head.

10. Stimulating the back of the throat while suctioning could result in:
    A. tachypnea.
    B. bronchospasm.
    C. bradypnea.
    D. bradycardia.

11. When you are preparing to suction the nasopharynx with a French catheter, determine its length by:
    A. measuring from the tip of the patient's nose to the angle of the jaw.
    B. measuring from the corner of the patient's mouth to the tip of the ear.
    C. measuring from the tip of the patient's nose to the tip of the ear.
    D. measuring from the corner of the patient's mouth to the angle of the jaw.

12. After inserting an oropharyngeal airway (OPA), the patient begins to gag. You should:
    A. insert a nasopharyngeal airway in addition to the oropharyngeal airway.
    B. immediately remove the oropharyngeal airway and prepare to suction.
    C. reassure the patient that the oropharyngeal airway is necessary.
    D. Ask the patient to breath deeply; the gagging will subside.

13. You have determined that the number of patients has exceeded your ability to effectively handle a scene and have summoned additional resources. Your next action should be to:
    A. move all patients to the transport area.
    B. immediately begin treating the patients.
    C. perform a focused history on the patients.
    D. triage the patients.

14. Which of the following best describes a deeply unresponsive patient?
    A. may have an intact gag reflex
    B. responds to tactile stimulation
    C. may cough when an airway adjunct is placed
    D. does not respond to pain

15. Which upper respiratory sound could indicate a liquid substance in the airway?
    A. crowing
    B. snoring
    C. gurgling
    D. stridor

16. You find that the patient's skin is pale, cool, and moist. You should suspect:
    A. hyperthermia.
    B. hypoperfusion.
    C. vasogenic shock.
    D. dehydration.

17. Which of the following would *not* be managed during the primary assessment?
    A. inadequate breathing.
    B. open chest injury.
    C. closed humerus fracture.
    D. major bleeding.

18. The purpose of performing a rapid trauma assessment is to
    A. assess a specific injury site.
    B. obtain accurate vital signs.
    C. obtain a SAMPLE history from the patient or bystanders.
    D. identify and manage life-threatening injuries.

19. When should the rapid trauma assessment be performed?
    A. while en route to the hospital on an unstable patient following vital sign assessment
    B. on the stable trauma patient after the ongoing assessment
    C. prior to moving the patient
    D. just before an unstable patient's arrival at the hospital

20. A major decision point for determining the sequence of assessment steps in the medical patient is:
    A. the patient's blood pressure.
    B. the patient's level of consciousness.
    C. the patient's respiratory status.
    D. the patient's pulse rate.

21. Having the patient rate his pain on a scale of 1 to 10 is assessing the
    A. radiation.
    B. quality.
    C. severity.
    D. provocation.

22. You are assessing a patient who complains of pelvic pain after a fall from a ladder. How would you assess the pelvis?
    A. Visually inspect it only.
    B. Rock the pelvis, checking for instability.
    C. Compress inward and downward.
    D. Apply firm pressure to the pubic bone.

23. A patient presents with a cough and states that he has been coughing up mucous. This is known as what type of cough?
    A. mucous
    B. rhonchi
    C. productive
    D. chronic

24. Palpation of the pelvic area in a trauma patient should be:
    A. omitted in the patient with pelvic pain.
    B. performed in the patient with pelvic pain.
    C. always performed with suspected injury.
    D. omitted if the patient is unresponsive.

25. The dorsalis pedis pulse is located:
    A. behind the inner ankle bone.
    B. at the bend of the elbow.
    C. behind the knee.
    D. on the top surface of the foot.

26. The first step in the ongoing assessment is to:
    A. check your interventions.
    B. repeat the focused assessment for other injuries or complaints.
    C. reassess and record vital signs.
    D. repeat the primary assessment.

27. You note a change in the patient's mental status during transport. You should immediately:
    A. take a complete set of vital signs.
    B. assess the effectiveness of emergency care.
    C. increase the patient's oxygenation.
    D. repeat the primary assessment.

28. Which of the following signs found during the ongoing assessment of an adult would indicate that the patient's condition is improving?
    A. The patient's breathing was bradypneic and is now tachypneic.
    B. The patient's skin color changes from cyanotic to blue-gray.
    C. The patient begins to use accessory muscles to breathe.
    D. The patient's heart rate increases from 40 beats/minute to 100.

29. How often should the ongoing assessment be repeated in the unstable patient?
    A. 2 minutes
    B. 3 minutes
    C. 4 minutes
    D. 5 minutes

QUESTIONS: 20–36 ■ 203

30. When you are dealing with a patient who seems hostile or aggressive, it could be necessary to assert your authority. Which position is likely to convey authority?
    A. Keep your eye level below the patient's.
    B. Keep your eye level above the patient's.
    C. Communicate without making eye contact.
    D. Communicate while staring at the patient.

31. After you have made numerous attempts to persuade a patient to be treated and transported, the patient refuses both, as well as to sign the refusal-of-care form. You should:
    A. force the patient to sign the form by refusing to leave until it is signed.
    B. have a family member sign the form to verify that the patient refused to sign it.
    C. leave the scene without the signature and advise dispatch of the situation.
    D. sign the patient's name for him and document the unusual circumstances.

32. Which of the following would *not* be considered a sign of *inadequate* breathing?
    A. restlessness and agitation
    B. acute abdominal pain
    C. accessory muscle use
    D. incomprehensible speech

33. When providing emergency care for the adult patient with breathing difficulty, you should:
    A. take time to determine the exact cause of the patient's distress.
    B. expose and inspect the chest in the trauma patient.
    C. provide positive pressure ventilation only if you are certain of the need.
    D. consider the patient who is responsive as a low treatment priority.

34. If you note a decrease in wheezing upon auscultation and a decrease in the mental status in a patient complaining of breathing difficulty, you should suspect that:
    A. the patient is definitely improving.
    B. the carbon dioxide levels have decreased.
    C. the breathing is improving since the patient is relaxing.
    D. the bronchoconstriction has worsened.

35. What effect would increased oxygenation have on a breathing patient's mental status?
    A. It generally causes no difference in the mental status.
    B. It causes the patient to become sleepy and drowsy.
    C. It can reduce the restlessness and anxiety.
    D. It causes dizziness and nausea.

36. During your primary assessment of a patient complaining of difficulty breathing, you note that the pulse is 140 beats/minute and the patient's neck is cyanotic. In what sequence should you perform your assessment and emergency care?
    A. Provide positive pressure ventilation, transport expeditiously, and continue assessment.
    B. Apply high-flow oxygen, continue the assessment, and transport to the hospital.
    C. Complete the physical assessment, apply positive pressure ventilation, and transport.
    D. Continue assessment, apply high-flow oxygen, call for advanced life support (ALS) backup, and transport.

37. You are treating a patient who is complaining of shortness of breath. The patient has minimal rise of the chest. You feel little airflow from the patient's mouth and nose. You should immediately:
    A. begin bag-valve-mask ventilation.
    B. provide oxygen by nonrebreather mask.
    C. apply a nasal cannula at 6 lpm.
    D. perform a detailed physical exam of the chest.

38. When assisting a patient with the administration of a bronchodilator by metered-dose inhaler, you should:
    A. not shake the canister because doing so disrupts the drug's effectiveness.
    B. have the patient exhale forcefully and rapidly after inhaling of the drug.
    C. instruct the patient to breathe out against pursed lips.
    D. depress the canister 1 to 2 seconds prior to the patient's inhalation.

39. Which condition could improve when a child is exposed to the cool night air?
    A. epiglottis
    B. croup
    C. asthma
    D. pulmonary embolism

40. The most common cause of mechanical failure associated with the automated external defibrillator is:
    A. cable breakage.
    B. 80 cycle interference.
    C. battery failure.
    D. cold temperature.

41. You respond to the scene for a patient in cardiac arrest. Upon arrival, the patient is pulseless and apneic. The family states that he went into cardiac arrest about 4 minutes prior to your arrival. You should immediately:

A. insert an oropharyngeal airway.
B. begin bag-valve-mask ventilation.
C. attach the automated external defibrillator (AED) and analyze the rhythm.
D. perform five cycles of CPR.

42. For which of the following patients would the administration of nitroglycerin be *inappropriate?*
    A. 52-year-old who has taken four nitroglycerin tablets before your arrival
    B. 77-year-old with a blood pressure of 110/64, pulse 90 beats/minute
    C. 62-year-old who continues to complain of chest pain after taking two nitroglycerin tablets
    D. 88-year-old who has taken one nitroglycerin tablet and now complains of a headache

43. A common side effect of nitroglycerin is:
    A. diaphoresis.
    B. bradycardia.
    C. hypotension.
    D. dyspnea.

44. To achieve the same dose as one nitroglycerin tablet, you would need to depress the nitroglycerin spray container how many times?
    A. once, delivering one short spray
    B. twice, delivering two short sprays
    C. three times, delivering one continuous spray
    D. once but hold the container down, delivering one continuous extended spray

45. The number one cause of death in the United States is:
    A. automobile accidents.
    B. falls.
    C. cancer.
    D. heart disease.

46. A patient experiencing a heart attack without chest pain or chest discomfort is said to be having a:
    A. silent heart attack.
    B. phantom heart attack.
    C. quiet heart attack.
    D. minor heart attack.

47. When applying the pads of an automated external defibrillator (AED) to the patient's chest, you notice a nitroglycerin patch on him. You should:
    A. place the adhesive defibrillation pad over the nitroglycerin patch.
    B. leave the patch in place and adhere the defibrillation pad immediately next to it.
    C. remove the nitroglycerin patch and wipe the area clean.
    D. move the AED pad to another location to avoid the patch.

48. The two basic categories of external defibrillators are the:
    A. automatic and semiautomatic.
    B. automatic and implantable.
    C. automatic and manual.
    D. manual and implantable.

49. After you have successfully defibrillated a patient, he has a strong radial pulse, but his breathing is shallow and slow. You should:
    A. wait until the respiratory drive returns and resumes the spontaneous respirations.
    B. apply a nasal cannula with the setting at 6 lpm.
    C. administer oxygen by nonrebreather mask at 15 lpm.
    D. begin bag-valve-mask ventilation at a rate of 10 to 12/minute.

50. Following the administration of nitroglycerin, it could:
    A. cause a slight increase in the patient's pulse rate.
    B. result in an increase in the patient's blood pressure.
    C. result in sudden and intense diarrhea and nausea.
    D. increase the heart's workload.

51. The ratio of chest compressions to ventilation in two-person CPR for an adult patient is:
    A. 5 compressions to 1 ventilation.
    B. 10 compressions to 1 ventilation.
    C. 15 compressions to 2 ventilations.
    D. 30 compressions to 2 ventilations.

52. The condition in which there is a lack of insulin and a high level of sugar in the blood is called:
    A. hypoglycemia.
    B. insulin shock.
    C. hypoinsulin.
    D. hyperglycemia.

53. In which position should you place a hypoglycemic patient who has an altered mental status?
    A. supine
    B. semi-Fowler
    C. Trendelenburg
    D. on the patient's side

54. Which symptom is a late sign of stroke?
    A. double vision
    B. stiff neck
    C. headache
    D. garbled speech

55. The *recovery phase* of a seizure in which the patient's mental status progressively improves over time is known as the:
    A. aura period.
    B. tonic phase.
    C. clonic phase.
    D. postictal state.

56. The stage of a generalized seizure during which the muscles become rigid is known as the:
    A. aura phase.
    B. tonic phase.
    C. clonic phase.
    D. postictal phase.

57. The symptoms associated with a transient ischemic attack generally subside within:
    A. 5 to 10 minutes.
    B. 30 minutes.
    C. 1 hour.
    D. 36 hours.

58. A major contributing factor to a stroke is:
    A. recent exercise.
    B. fever.
    C. high blood pressure.
    D. seizure.

59. A condition in which the patient has a sudden and temporary loss of consciousness is called:
    A. neuropoxia.
    B. syncope.
    C. postictal.
    D. eclampsia.

60. Which signs and symptoms most likely indicate an allergic reaction?
    A. headache and restlessness
    B. respiratory distress and shock

C. runny and watery eyes
D. general weakness and abdominal cramping

61. You have just administered epinephrine by autoinjector to a patient having an anaphylactic reaction to a bee sting. How long would you expect the drug to be effective?
    A. 10 to 20 minutes
    B. 30 to 40 minutes
    C. 50 to 60 minutes
    D. 2 to 3 hours

62. A 65-year-old patient is suffering from a mild allergic reaction. There are no signs of respiratory compromise or shock. You should:
    A. inject one-half of the adult dose of epinephrine via an autoinjector.
    B. administer one-fourth of the adult dose of epinephrine via an autoinjector.
    C. withhold epinephrine at any dose unless medical direction provides for its administration.
    D. administer a full adult dose of epinephrine via an autoinjector.

63. A substance that triggers an allergic reaction is called:
    A. an allergen.
    B. a parasite.
    C. an access particle.
    D. an antibody.

64. Activated charcoal can be used in ingested poisonings because it:
    A. inhibits poisons from being absorbed into the body.
    B. neutralizes poisons while in the stomach and gastrointestinal tract.
    C. prevents poisons from entering the cells by neutralization.
    D. acts as an antidote to most household and commercial poisons.

65. In which position should the patient complaining of an acute abdomen with signs of hypoperfusion be placed?
    A. left lateral recumbent
    B. supine with feet elevated
    C. semi-Fowler with knees bent
    D. position of comfort

66. Which of the following persons would likely tolerate a cold environment best and have a reduced risk of hypothermia?
    A. a three-year-old child who is wet from a rain shower
    B. a 20-year-old person who has been drinking alcohol
    C. a 34-year-old person who has been walking in a stiff wind
    D. a 50-year-old person who takes blood pressure medication

67. When treating a patient who has been bitten by a rattlesnake, you should:
    A. wash the area around the bite with mild soap and water.
    B. elevate the injection site above the level of the patient's heart.
    C. make two small lacerations over the bite and evacuate the wound.
    D. place a tourniquet superior and inferior to the bite injection site.

68. *Reasonable force* is defined as the:
    A. use of moderate force to control a dangerous patient who you have determined is a risk.
    B. amount of force needed to overpower and restrain an unruly patient who could injure others.
    C. use of physical and tactile force to subdue a patient and prevent injury to all concerned.
    D. minimal amount of force required to keep the patient from injuring himself or others.

69. Which position will help reduce the risk of supine hypotension syndrome in the patient who is near full term of her pregnancy?
    A. prone
    B. shock
    C. supine
    D. lateral recumbent

70. Which statement pertaining to the normal delivery of an infant is correct?
    A. The placenta most often is delivered 1 to 2 hours after birth.
    B. Gentle pressure should be applied to the fontanel during delivery.
    C. Bleeding after delivery can be up to 1,000 cc and is well tolerated.
    D. The placenta must be transported to the hospital for examination.

71. When treating a patient who has just delivered a baby in the prehospital setting, you should
    A. apply traction to the cord to aid delivery of placenta.
    B. transport without delay and allow the placenta to deliver while en route.
    C. delay transport until the placenta has been completely delivered.
    D. place the mother in a Fowler's position to make her more comfortable.

72. The umbilical cord should be cut:
    A. as soon after delivery as possible.
    B. after the cord pulsations cease.
    C. before cord pulsations cease.
    D. after the single clamp has been placed.

73. During delivery, the gloved fingertips are positioned on the bony part of the infant's head to:
    A. delay delivery until arrival at the hospital.
    B. prevent an explosive delivery of the head.
    C. slow delivery until arrival at the hospital.
    D. monitor the infant's pulse rate during labor.

74. Your patient has a deep laceration to the upper arm with bright red blood spurting from the wound. Which vessel is likely severed?
    A. brachial artery
    B. femoral artery
    C. cephalic vein
    D. peroneal vein

75. Your patient was involved in an industrial accident and is bleeding dark red blood profusely from the leg. During which assessment phase should you initially control this patient's bleeding?
    A. focused history and physical exam
    B. detailed physical exam
    C. primary assessment
    D. ongoing assessment

76. Your patient has sustained a large hematoma from an accident on the playground. How should you proceed with your emergency care for the closed soft tissue injury?
    A. Ensure airway and breathing, splint any injuries, take body substance isolation precautions, and treat shock.
    B. Ensure airway and breathing, take book substance isolation (BSI) precautions, splint any injuries, and treat shock.
    C. Take book substance isolation (BSI) precautions, ensure airway and breathing, treat shock, and splint any injuries.
    D. Take book substance isolation (BSI) precautions, treat shock, ensure airway and breathing, and splint any injuries.

77. While removing a burn patient's clothing, you find that a portion of the shirt has adhered to the patient's back. You should:
    A. gently remove clothing from the adhered area by pulling.
    B. cut the shirt off around the adhered portion.
    C. apply a burn ointment to the adhered area.
    D. soak the adhered area with water and then remove adhered clothing.

78. Which of the following is *inappropriate* treatment for a patient suffering from burns?
    A. Cover the patient to prevent body heat loss.
    B. Separate burned fingers with dry dressings.
    C. Stop the burning process by applying water.
    D. Attempt to drain blisters by applying direct pressure.

79. A bandage is designed to:
    A. hold a dressing in place.
    B. be sterile or free from any organisms.
    C. be removed if bleeding is not controlled.
    D. go directly cover an open wound and prevent infection.

80. Blood has soaked through the pressure dressing you applied to your patient's injury. You should immediately:
    A. apply a loose tourniquet until you can feel a pulse.
    B. apply a tight tourniquet because the bleeding is uncontrollable.
    C. remove the original dressings and then apply new ones.
    D. apply additional dressings over the original ones.

81. Why should you leave the fingertips or toes exposed after bandaging an extremity?
    A. It provides for patient comfort through temperature control.
    B. It eliminates the potential for circulatory obstruction.
    C. It allows for rapid removal of bandages if required.
    D. It allows for the assessment of circulation.

82. Your patient has a knife embedded in the right side of his chest. You should immediately:
    A. expose the wound area.
    B. control wound bleeding.
    C. gently remove the object.
    D. manually secure the object.

83. The anterior bone of the lower leg is called the:
    A. fibula.
    B. ulna.
    C. tibia.
    D. femur.

84. When providing emergency care for a patient with an isolated fracture, you should:
    A. make three attempts to align a fracture if the distal pulses are absent.
    B. pad the splint to prevent pressure and discomfort to the patient.
    C. leave all jewelry in place to prevent accusations of stealing if any are lost.
    D. retract the protruding bones back beneath the skin to reduce the incidence of infection.

85. When assessing a potential spine-injured patient, you should:
    A. ask the patient to move any painful areas to determine the specific area of injury.
    B. not suspect spine injury if the patient has adequate breathing.
    C. check the sensory function only in the extremities so the patient does not move.
    D. assess the motor and sensory functions before and after the patient is secured to a backboard.

86. You should leave a motorcycle helmet in place if:
    A. it interferes with your ability to assess the airway and breathing.
    B. it interferes with your ability to manage the airway and breathing.
    C. it does not fit well and allows excessive movement of the head.
    D. you can properly immobilize the spine with the helmet in place.

87. When providing care for chemical burns to the eye, you should:
    A. postpone flushing of the eyes until transport has begun.
    B. flush alkali burns with vinegar for at least 10 minutes.
    C. flush the eyes immediately and continue during transport.
    D. be certain never to remove hard or soft contact lenses.

88. Which of the following signs and symptoms indicates that a pediatric patient is in decompensated respiratory failure?
    A. cyanosis
    B. nasal flaring
    C. subcostal retractions
    D. increased respiratory rate

89. Which of the following signs or symptoms is the best indication of hypoperfusion (shock) in the pediatric patient?
    A. noisy respiration
    B. weak or absent peripheral pulse
    C. pink, warm, and dry skin
    D. capillary refill in less than 2 seconds

90. The failure of a caregiver to provide sufficient attention or respect to an individual, is called:
    A. abuse.
    B. neglect.
    C. molestation.
    D. violation.

91. Which action is considered dangerous when navigating a curve while driving the ambulance?
    A. entering the curve on the outside
    B. braking prior to entering the curve
    C. decelerating before entering the curve
    D. accelerating while in the curve

92. To protect yourself and the patient during the extrication process from debris such as glass and metal, you should:
    A. direct the hydraulic spreader operator to be careful.
    B. quickly perform a rapid extrication procedure.
    C. cover the patient and yourself with a tarpaulin.
    D. remove your heavy coat and cover the patient.

93. Which of the following best describes simple access to a patient?
    A. access that takes less than 20 minutes
    B. access that does not require the use of tools
    C. access that requires special training
    D. access gained by using a manually forced tool

94. You are approaching a motor vehicle crash site and notice a truck overturned with a plume of yellow gas surrounding the site. Your first action should be to:
    A. cordon off the area and evacuate all bystanders from the area.
    B. approach the site slowly in an attempt to identify the cargo.

C. approach the site quickly and remove any injured patients.
    D. assist bystanders to an area downhill and downwind of the site.

95. You are the first to arrive on a scene of a mass casualty incident (MCI). What is your initial role as the first EMT on the scene?
    A. treatment manager
    B. incident manager
    C. triage officer
    D. staging sector

96. You are at the scene of a multiple casualty incident and have been assigned to the triage sector. Your patient has sustained a large burn without airway complications. You would prioritize this patient as:
    A. red—high priority.
    B. yellow—second priority.
    C. green—low priority.
    D. black—lowest priority.

97. Placement of a nasogastric tube is indicated for a child when:
    A. an endotracheal tube can be placed within 30 seconds.
    B. the responsive patient is developing gastric distention.
    C. effective ventilations are prevented due to gastric distention.
    D. the responsive patient is at risk of vomiting.

98. A piece of equipment that could be needed specifically when performing endotracheal intubation is:
    A. a stylet.
    B. a mask.
    C. oxygen tubing.
    D. oxygen flow meter.

99. During endotracheal intubation, the stylet is used to:

    A. facilitate suctioning of the endotracheal tube.
    B. secure the endotracheal tube in place.
    C. alter the shape of the endotracheal tube and provide stiffness.
    D. remove an improperly positioned endotracheal tube.

100. The *least* critical of the common complication that can occur with endotracheal intubation is:

    A. hypoxia from the interruption of ventilation.
    B. left mainstem intubation.
    C. trauma to the lips, tongue, or teeth.
    D. bradycardia during laryngoscopy.

101. Touching or stimulating the epiglottis or vocal cords during intubation can result in:

    A. acute laryngospasm.
    B. endotracheal swelling.
    C. aspiration due to vomiting.
    D. loss of tube sterility.

102. During intubation attempts in the infant, the presence of bradycardia can indicate:

    A. the need for nasogastric tube placement.
    B. correct tube placement.
    C. hypoxia.
    D. gastric distention.

103. Placement of an endotracheal tube by using the fingers of one hand is called:

    A. digital intubation.
    B. manual intubation.
    C. fingertip intubation.
    D. oral intubation.

Scenario

Questions 104 to 106 refer to the following scenario:

You arrive on the scene and find a 32-year-old male patient who the police claim was stabbed in the chest following an altercation in a parking lot. Upon your arrival at the scene, the police are present and have the perpetrator in custody. You find the patient lying supine and fully clothed. He moans when you apply painful stimuli. The first responders on the scene indicate that his airway is clear and his breathing is 42/minute and shallow. His radial pulse is rapid but strong. His skin is slightly pale, cool, and clammy. His face is cyanotic. He has a stab wound to the left lateral chest at the 4th intercostal space. His blood pressure is 112/62 mmHg. His SpO_2 is 82 percent.

104. What should be your next immediate action?

    A. Apply a nonrebreather mask at 15 lpm and prepare the patient for transport.
    B. Obtain a set of vital signs.
    C. Attempt to get a SAMPLE history from the patient.
    D. Occlude the open wound with your gloved hand.

105. The vital signs indicate the patient is most likely experiencing:

    A. severe bleeding and hypovolemic shock.
    B. inadequate oxygen exchange and hypoxia.
    C. a head injury.
    D. a spinal injury.

106. The next step in your emergency care should be to:

    A. apply a nasal cannula at 6 lpm.
    B. begin immediate transport.
    C. begin bag-valve-mask ventilation.
    D. administer oxygen via a nonrebreather mask.

107. You have responded to a car stalled in swift water from a torrential rainstorm. The water has risen to the bottom of the windows and appears to be moving rapidly. Your patient has crawled to the roof of the vehicle and is waving his arms and pleading for help. You should:
    A. call for a specialized swift water rescue team and wait for its arrival.
    B. carefully try to reach the patient by wading out to the vehicle.
    C. call for a backup EMS unit to coordinate the rescue attempt.
    D. throw a rope to the patient so he can be pulled to safety.

108. A patient has suffered an injury to the left leg just above the patella. The leg is angulated and the bone is protruding through the skin. Which of the following best describes this injury and how it should be documented on the patient care report?
    A. retracted fracture to the right proximal tibia
    B. closed fracture to the right distal femur
    C. compound fracture to the left proximal tibia
    D. open fracture to the left distal femur

109. You are assessing a 43-year-old patient with a 4 centimeter laceration to the left arm. The bleeding is dark red and flows steadily from the wound. You would suspect that the source of bleeding is:
    A. capillary.
    B. arteriole.
    C. venous.
    D. arterial.

110. Your patient presents with a large wound to her right lower leg, which is bleeding profusely. There is no deformity of the extremity. After taking appropriate body substance isolation precautions, your next immediate step in emergency care of the patient is to:
    A. apply a tourniquet.
    B. use a pressure point.
    C. apply direct pressure.
    D. elevate the extremity.

111. Upon arrival at the scene, you find an unresponsive 34-year-old male who has sustained a large wound to the frontal portion of his head. Your partner immediately applies direct pressure to the wound. The patient is breathing at 32 breaths per minute with shallow rise of the chest. You note gurgling on inspiration and exhalation. His radial pulse is 42 beats/minute. You should immediately:
    A. administer oxygen via a nonrebreather mask.
    B. begin bag-valve-mask ventilation.
    C. begin chest compressions.
    D. suction the airway.

112. You arrive on the scene and find a 26-year-old male patient with a gunshot wound to the right anterior chest wall. Your partner applies an occlusive dressing to the wound. The vital signs are blood pressure, 72/52 mmHg; heart rate, 52 beats/minute; respiration, 16 with adequate chest rise; also, the skin is flushed, warm, and dry, SpO_2 is 99 percent while on a nonrebreather mask. You should suspect:
    A. massive blood loss with hypovolemic shock.
    B. spinal injury with distributive shock.
    C. large pneumothorax to the right lung.
    D. head injury with an increase in intracranial pressure.

113. A patient has sustained a superficial partial thickness burn from touching a hot exhaust pipe. This is an example of what type of burn?
    A. arc
    B. radiant
    C. flash
    D. contact

114. You are treating a 12-year-old patient who has a suspected fracture of the right hand that he sustained when he fell off his skateboard. You should:
    A. place a roll of bandage in the patient's hand and extend the fingers when splinting.
    B. extend the hand and curl the fingers to the underside of the splint.
    C. secure the hand to the splint with the palm facing in an upward position.
    D. splint the hand with the fist in a tightly clenched position.

115. To best monitor improvement or deterioration of the head injury, you should obtain a series of:
    A. Cincinnati Prehospital Stroke Scale scores.
    B. vital signs.
    C. Los Angeles Prehospital Stroke Scale scores.
    D. Glasgow Coma Scale scores.

116. In what position should an unresponsive medical patient who requires ventilation be placed?
    A. supine
    B. lateral recumbent
    C. Fowler's
    D. Trendelenburg

117. You are the second unit to arrive at an industrial accident that has amputated the patient's right arm from the shoulder. The first unit transported the patient while the severed arm was being disentangled from the machinery. To transport the amputated arm, you should:
    A. wrap it in a dry, sterile dressing and put in a plastic bag with ice.
    B. wrap it in a dry, sterile dressing, cover it with an occlusive dressing, and place it on ice.
    C. wrap it in a saline-moistened, sterile dressing and cover it with ice.
    D. wrap it in a saline-moistened, sterile dressing, put it in a plastic bag, and keep it cool.

118. You have responded to a motor vehicle crash that involves two vehicles with moderate damage. The patients are still in the vehicles and are alert. In an attempt to minimize any further risk from the vehicles, you should immediately:
    A. disconnect the battery cables.
    B. pull all of the fuses.
    C. disconnect the spark plug wires.
    D. turn off the ignition.

119. The best emergency care for an abdominal evisceration is to cover the exposed organs with:
    A. a sterile dressing moistened with saline and then an occlusive dressing.
    B. an occlusive dressing and then a sterile gauze moistened with saline.
    C. a dry, sterile cotton dressing and then an occlusive dressing.
    D. a sterile dressing covered in sterile water or sterile saline.

120. Upon arrival at the scene, you find a 17-year-old patient who fell while rock climbing. He is not alert as you approach him. You hear sonorous sounds. You should immediately:
    A. suction the airway.
    B. insert an oropharyngeal airway.
    C. establish manual inline spine stabilization.
    D. open the airway with a jaw-thrust maneuver.

121. You arrive at a local boat dock for a patient with an eye injury. You find a 23-year-old male who sustained a laceration to his eyelid from a fishing hook. The fishing hook avulsed a portion of the eyelid but has not penetrated the eye. You should manage the eyelid injury by:
    A. covering the eye with a dry sterile dressing.
    B. applying direct pressure to the eyelid and eyeball to control any bleeding.
    C. apply an antibacterial ointment to prevent an eye infection.
    D. cover the eye with a moist, sterile dressing.

122. You would most likley suspect a tension pneumothorax if the patient presented with absent:
    A. breath sounds on the uninjured side and decreased breath sounds on the injured side.
    B. breath sounds at the lower lobes and decreased breath sounds at the upper lobes.
    C. breath sounds on the injured side and decreased breath sounds on the uninjured side.
    D. breath sounds in the upper lobes and decreased breath sounds in the lower lobes of the lungs.

123. While assessing a patient who has suffered a head injury, you find blood-tinged fluid flowing freely from his right ear. You should:
    A. carefully pack the ear with a dressing.
    B. swab the inside of the ear with a cotton swab.
    C. apply direct pressure by placing a balled up dressing in the ear.
    D. place a loose dressing across the opening of the ear.

124. Upon arrival, you find an 83-year-old female patient who is complaining of severe shortness of breath, weakness, and fatigue. Her vital signs are blood pressure, 198/102 mmHg; heart rate, 134 beats/minute; respiration, 28 with accessory muscle use; and pulse oximeter reading of 82 percent. The skin is pale, cool, and clammy. You hear crackle/rales throughout the lungs on auscultation. The patient has a history of congestive heart failure. You should immediately:
    A. insert an oropharyngeal airway.
    B. apply a nonrebreather mask at 15 lpm.
    C. begin bag-valve-mask ventilation.
    D. administer one nitroglycerin tablet.

125. You arrive on the scene and find an alert 73-year-old male patient in his recliner. The patient suddenly was unable to get out of the recliner after eating lunch. His vital signs are blood pressure, 186/98 mmHg; heart rate, 82 beats/minute and irregular; respiration, 20/minute with good chest rise; and pulse oximeter reading is 95 percent on room air. The skin is warm and dry. He has severe numbness to his left arm and slurred speech. You should suspect he is having:
    A. a silent heart attack.
    B. a stroke.
    C. an anaphylactic reaction.
    D. a drug reaction.

126. The most reliable assessment findings to determine whether a patient is having a stroke are:
    A. blood pressure and heart rate.
    B. mental status and baseline vital signs.
    C. arm strength, facial droop, and speech.
    D. pulse oximetry and respiratory rate.

127. You arrive on the scene and find a patient who had a syncopal episode. The patient states that the syncope came on suddenly with no warning. The patient is also complaining of discomfort in his chest. You should next immediately:
    A. apply a nonrebreather mask and administer one nitroglycerin tablet.
    B. place the patient on the cot and begin rapid transport.
    C. administer one nitroglycerin tablet and then assess the blood pressure.
    D. apply a nasal cannula and assess the patient's circulation.

128. You arrive on the scene and find a 14-year-old male patient who is complaining of severe shortness of breath. Upon assessment, you find that he is hoarse and has stridor on inhalation. His breathing is labored at 28 times/minute. His skin is warm, red, and blotchy. His radial pulse is 132 per minute. You would suspect that this patient is suffering from:
    A. hypoglycemia.
    B. diabetic ketoacidosis
    C. an allergic reaction.
    D. a syncopal episode.

129. A four-year-old patient is experiencing breathing difficulty. While enroute to the hospital, the patient is seated on his mother's lap. You attempt to place a nonrebreather mask on the child, but he will not tolerate it. Your next action should be to:
    A. have the patient's mother forcibly hold the mask over the child's face.
    B. have the patient's mother hold the mask near the child's face.
    C. take the child from the mother and hold the mask over the child's face.
    D. discontinue your efforts to apply oxygen to the child.

130. A large number of patients who have been successfully defibrillated will:
    A. deteriorate back into ventricular fibrillation.
    B. remain apneic for at least 24 hours.
    C. require at least one more defibrillation once the pulse has been regained.
    D. not require any additional treatment or transport to a medical facility.

131. You arrive on the scene and find a 68-year-old female patient complaining of chest discomfort and shortness of breath. Suddenly, she slumps forward. Upon your primary assessment, you find she is apneic and has no radial or carotid pulse. Your next immediate action is to:
    A. begin a rapid medical assessment to determine the cause of the unresponsiveness.
    B. initiate bag-valve-mask ventilation once an oropharyngeal airway has been inserted.
    C. apply the automated external defibrillator and initiate the rhythm analysis.
    D. begin five cycles of CPR and then attach the automated external defibrillator and analyze the rhythm.

132. You apply an automated external defibrillator (AED) to a patient, and it indicates a shock. You suspect the patient is in what rhythm?
    A. atrial fibrillation
    B. asystole
    C. ventricular fibrillation
    D. pulseless electrical activity

133. You arrive on the scene and find a 27-year-old male patient in the second floor bathroom of his home. He is alert but responding inappropriately to your questions. His breathing is a normal volume at 22/minute. His radial pulse is 113/minute and the skin is pale, cool, and clammy. His blood pressure is 128/76 mmHg, and his pulse oximeter reading is 98 percent. When asked about medications, a family member brings you a vial of Humulin that is cold. You conduct a rapid medical assessment and find no evidence of trauma or any other signs or symptoms. Your next immediate action should be to:

    A. administer one tube of oral glucose.
    B. apply a nasal cannula at 6 lpm.
    C. perform a detailed physical exam.
    D. administer 0.30 mg of epinephrine.

134. An early sign of hypoxia in a patient exhibiting respiratory distress is:

    A. bradycardia.
    B. tachypnea.
    C. intercostal retractions.
    D. agitation and restlessness.

135. You arrive on the scene of a patient who is actively seizing. He suffered one seizure prior to your arrival and did not regain responsiveness before he seized the second time. He has been seizing for approximately 15 minutes. The patient has a history of diabetes mellitus and epilepsy. You should:

    A. guide the patient's movements so that he does not injure himself.
    B. immediately insert an oropharyngeal airway and begin bag-valve-mask ventilation.
    C. administer one tube of oral glucose and contact advanced life support.
    D. restrain the patient onto a backboard and quickly move him into the ambulance.

136. You arrive on the scene and find a 62-year-old male patient complaining of chest discomfort. His respiratory rate is 18/minute with a good tidal volume. His radial pulse is weak. His skin is pale, cool, and clammy. His blood pressure is 136/88 mmHg. He has a prescription for nitroglycerin. You should immediately:

    A. administer one nitroglycerin tablet sublingually.
    B. assess his blood pressure again to determine whether nitroglycerin can be administered.
    C. place the patient in left lateral recumbent position.
    D. apply a nasal cannula at 2 to 4 lpm.

137. Your patient is experiencing an anaphylactic reaction. The skin is warm and red due to:

    A. vasoconstriction.
    B. bronchoconstriciton.
    C. decreased capillary permeability.
    D. systemic vasodilation.

138. You arrive on the scene and find a 58-year-old female patient lying supine on the living room couch. Her husband greets you at the door and indicates that his wife has been complaining of chest discomfort for about three hours. You approach the patient and find that she is not alert or responding to your voice. She does not respond to a pinch to the web of her hand. You should immediately:

    A. apply a nonrebreather mask at 15 lpm and assess the carotid pulse.
    B. perform a head-tilt, chin-lift maneuver and assess the respirations.
    C. apply the automated external defibrillator and begin the rhythm analysis.
    D. administer one tube of oral glucose.

139. Upon assessing a suspected stroke patient, you note that the patient is unable to feel you lightly touching her left foot. You would note this as:
   A. a neurological deficit.
   B. a normal finding.
   C. an indication of the involvement of the spinal cord.
   D. a side effect of severe systolic hypertension.

140. You arrive on the scene and find a patient with a history of diabetes mellitus who is not responding to verbal stimuli. His airway is open, and he is breathing at 18/minute with shallow chest rise. His radial pulse is strong at 104/minute. You should immediately:
   A. administer one dose of oral glucose and conduct an ongoing assessment.
   B. insert an oropharyngeal airway and begin bag-valve-mask ventilation.
   C. begin positive pressure ventilation and administer one tube of oral glucose.
   D. immediately prepare for transport and administer oral glucose while en route.

141. A convulsion is characterized as:
   A. a visual disturbance or unusual smell or sensation.
   B. contracted and tense muscles that do not relax.
   C. muscle rigidity that alternates with muscle relaxation.
   D. a period of confusion, fatigue, and headache.

142. The patient suffering a severe allergic reaction is likely to exhibit the following signs or symptoms:
   A. urticaria; pruritis; red, warm skin; tachycardia; and hypotension.
   B. pale, cool, clammy skin; decreased mental status; tachycardia; and hypotension.
   C. warm, dry skin; hypertension; bradycardia; and crackle/rales.
   D. muscular rigidity; fever; hypotension; and absent breath sounds on one side.

143. You are providing positive pressure ventilation to an unresponsive 60-year-old female. The patient's pulse rate continues to increase from 86/minute to 108/minute, yet she remains unresponsive. This is likely an indication of:
   A. an improvement in the oxygenation of the cells.
   B. a reduction in the amount of carbon dioxide.
   C. ineffective positive pressure ventilation.
   D. an overdose from a narcotic substance.

144. You are called to the scene for a patient who is complaining of shortness of breath. Upon your assessment, you find that the patient is alert, has a respiratory rate or 24 breaths/minute, and a radial pulse of 118/minute. Following your focused history and physical exam, you determine that he has bilateral wheezing. Your partner gathers multiple drugs from the night stand. You should consider administering which of the following medications from the nightstand?
   A. nitroglycerin
   B. ventolin
   C. coumadin
   D. digitalis

145. A patient who complains of a sudden onset of the "worst headache I have ever had" is most likely suffering from:
   A. an embolic stroke.
   B. hypoglycemia.
   C. a hemorrhagic stroke.
   D. a thrombotic stroke.

146. You arrive on the scene and find a 55-year-old male patient who has an obvious facial droop, right side paralysis, and slurred speech. As you are preparing to unload the patient out of the ambulance when you arrive at the hospital, you note that the patient's speech is normal and his face is no longer drooped. You would suspect the patient had:

    A. an embolic sroke.
    B. a transient ischemic attack.
    C. a thrombotic stroke.
    D. a hypoglycemic epidose.

147. You have administered an epinephrine autoinjector to the patient suffering from an anaphylactic reaction. During your second ongoing assessment, you note that the patient's breathing is still very labored with diffuse bilateral wheezing, the blood pressure is 78/54 mmHg, and the heart rate is 103/minute. You should next:

    A. contact medical direction for an order to administer benadryl.
    B. determine whether someone at the scene has a beta 2 metered-dose inhaler.
    C. administer a second epinephrine autoinjector if it is available.
    D. apply the automated external defibrillator in case the patient goes into cardiac arrest.

148. Insulin has which of the following effects?

    A. It allows glucose to enter the cell at a rate 10 times faster than without the glucose.
    B. It causes the liver to convert glycogen to glucose.
    C. It converts noncarbohydrate substances into glucose.
    D. It increases the blood glucose level by causing the production of glucose from glycogen.

149. During your SAMPLE history of a patient complaining of cardiac type chest pain, you note that the patient has a prescription for nitroglycerin. His vital signs are blood pressure, 138/76 mmHg; heart rate, 102 beats/minute; respiration 19 with good chest rise. The patient states that he took an aspirin, Sudaphed, and a Viagra pill within the last hour. You should:

    A. proceed with the administration of three nitroglycerin tablets.
    B. administer only one nitroglycerin and reassess the blood pressure.
    C. use only nitroglycerin spray under the tongue.
    D. not administer the nitroglycerin due to a contraindication.

150. You arrive on the scene and find a 23-year-old male patient who is complaining of dyspnea and numbness in his extremities. He was just held up at gunpoint at a local store. You conduct an assessment and find that he is not injured. He also states that his chest is tight and he feels lightheaded. His blood pressure is 148/88; heart rate is 103; and respiration rate is 36 and full. His breath sounds are clear bilaterally. You suspect that the patient is suffering from:

    A. hyperventilation syndrome.
    B. an acute asthma attack.
    C. angina pectoris.
    D. a myocardial infarction.

answers & rationales

1.
D. An example of an unsafe on-scene activity is entering a crime scene quickly before law enforcement has controlled the situation.

2.
B. People react to stress differently. Behavioral reactions include overeating, increased alcohol and drug use, teeth grinding, hyperactivity, or lack of energy. Choices A, C, and D are psychological reactions to stress. In addition to behavioral and psychological reactions, some people react socially (increased interpersonal conflicts) or cognitively, which includes confusion and loss of objectivity.

3.
D. The single most important way to prevent the spread of infection is by hand washing. Contaminants can be removed from the hands by 10 to 15 seconds of vigorous scrubbing with plain soap.

4.
C. As an EMT, you will be called to crime scenes or dangerous situations. Never enter a possibly dangerous scene; always position your vehicle away from it and wait for the police to stabilize the situation. Parking in view of the scene could endanger the EMS crew and escalate the anger of the people on the scene because you are not making patient contact. If you enter a scene and it then becomes hostile, quickly leave and wait for the police to arrive and secure it.

5.
C. Most states require EMT to report elder or child abuse, crimes, and drug-related injuries. Some states may require reporting of infectious disease exposure, use of patient restraints, mentally incompetent or intoxicated patients, attempted suicides, and dog bites.

6.
C. The anatomical term that means "on both sides" is *bilateral. Lateral* is toward the side or away from the mid-line. *Unilateral* means on one side. *Proximal* means near the point of reference.

7.
C. The ball and socket joint such as the shoulder permits the widest range of motion of all the joints. These joints permit flexion, extension, adduction, abduction and rotation. Another ball and socket joint is the hip. The pivot joint permits a turning motion; examples are the head, neck, and wrist. Gliding joints permit the sliding of one bone against another, such as those joints located in the hands and feet. Hinged joints permit flexion and extension; examples are those found in the elbow, fingers, and knee.

8.
B. Breathing may be slightly irregular when the patient sighs; this is a normal event that allows for deeper breaths to occur. The adult patient should be breathing between 12 to 20 times a minute. It is normal for a 6-month-old to breathe with the use of abdominal muscles; however, the rate should be between 25 and 50 times a minute. A patient breathing with the use of accessory muscles is in respiratory distress. The use of accessory muscles is an attempt to force more air into the lungs to relieve the shortness of breath. Unequal chest expansion is a sign of distress and could be caused by injury.

9.

A. Using a jaw-thrust maneuver will open the airway without compromising the spine. Use it when you suspect the possibility of a spinal injury. The head-tilt, chin-lift maneuver compromises the spine when opening the airway. This is a general distracter; however, you should never pull traction on the spine because this could lead to further injury. Tilting the head of a possibly spine-injured patient could injure him further. Open the airway by using the jaw-thrust maneuver.

10.

D. Stimulating the back of the throat while suctioning could result in bradycardia, a slowing of the heart. This area has sensitive nerves and if stimulated, they could cause a decrease in the heart rate, further complicating the patient's condition. *Bronchospasm* refers to the constriction of the bronchi; *tachypnea* is a fast breathing rate, and bradypnea is a slow breathing rate.

11.

C. The correct way to measure the length of catheter needed to suction the nasopharynx is from the tip of the patient's nose to the tip of the ear. Choices B and D are correct ways to measure the proper length of an oropharyngeal airway.

12.

B. If the patient begins to gag after the insertion of an OPA, you must immediately remove it, prepare to suction and insert a nasopharyngeal airway. The OPA can be used only in the completely unresponsive patient.

13.

D. You should first triage the patients. This helps to organize the emergency care they receive. Any critically injured patients should be treated before those with minor injuries. Treating and transporting patients in an organized manner will reduce on-scene time and increase the survival of the patients.

14.

D. An unresponsive patient who does not respond to pain will not cough or gag when an airway adjunct is placed into his throat.

15.

C. Liquid substances in the upper airway result in gurgling sounds. Crowing and stridor are produced on inspiration and are associated with upper airway swelling or muscle spasm. Snoring is caused by a partial airway obstruction of the tongue or epiglottis.

16.

B. The patient who presents with pale, cool, and moist skin is likely in a state of decreased perfusion (hypoperfusion). This state should clue you to look for the onset of shock. Hyperthermia, an elevated body core temperature, usually presents with hot, red skin. Vasogenic shock, which causes the vascular system to dilate, usually presents with red skin.

17.

C. Life threats that require immediate treatment during the primary assessment include airway control, breathing inadequacy, injuries to the chest, and major bleeding. Fracture management is a secondary injury and is not considered a life threat.

18.

D. When performing the rapid trauma assessment, which is based on the mechanism of injury, you are most concerned with identifying and managing life-threatening injuries. The specific injury site is assessed during the focused trauma assessment.

19.

C. The rapid trauma assessment is performed rapidly prior to moving the patient. The detailed physical exam is performed while transporting the patient. If other injuries are suspected when evaluating a stable trauma patient, always perform a rapid trauma assessment to determine whether other life-threatening injuries are present.

20.

B. The patient's level of consciousness is a major determining factor in the sequence of steps to take. If the patient is responsive, obtain the history and perform a focused medical assessment. If the patient is unresponsive, perform the rapid medical assessment followed by the history.

21.

C. Severity questions relate to how bad the pain is. Many patients can rate the pain on a scale from 1 to 10 with 10 being the worst. This method will help you when you reevaluate the patient. If the pain was originally a 4 but has increased to an 8, it has become worse.

22.

A. If a patient complains of pelvic pain, visually inspect it only. Palpating or manipulating the pelvis could cause further injury and severe pain. If the patient does *not* complain of pelvic pain or is unresponsive, palpate by placing both hands on the anterior lateral wings of the pelvis. When palpating the pelvis, you should use gentle inward and downward compression. Do not rock the pelvis or apply too much pressure.

23.

C. A productive cough is one that produces mucous. Note the color, consistency, and amount.

24.

A. Palpation of the pelvic region is omitted in a patient who is complaining of pelvic pain but should be performed in a patient who denies pain or is unresponsive.

25.

D. The dorsalis pedis pulse is located on the top surface of the foot. The posterior tibial pulse is located behind the inner anklebone. The brachial pulse is located at the bend of the elbow. The popliteal is located behind the knee.

26.

D. The first step in the ongoing assessment is to repeat the primary assessment. Follow this by reassessing and recording vital signs, repeating the focused assessment, and rechecking your interventions.

27.

D. If the patient's condition has worsened, you should first perform an ongoing assessment, which begins with a repeat of the primary assessment.

28.

D. The patient's heart rate was too slow (bradycardia) and is now 100 beats each minute, which is normal in the adult patient. It is not a sign of improvement when the patient who was breathing too slowly (bradypnea) is now breathing too fast (tachypnea). The patient's skin color is a good indication of the effectiveness of the oxygenation. A change from cyanotic to blue-gray is a sign of inadequate oxygenation and poor perfusion of the tissue. When a patient begins to use accessory muscles to breathe, he is deteriorating and needs to be ventilated with positive pressure ventilation.

29.

D. The primary assessment and the baseline vital signs should be repeated every 5 minutes in an unstable patient. Repeat every 15 minutes in the stable patient.

30.

B. Keeping your eye level above that of patient who is hostile or aggressive helps to assert your authority. This simple positioning can make a great deal of difference in the difficult patient. Positioning yourself below the patient's eye level can convey a submissive position. You should avoid staring at a patient; make eye contact just as you would in a normal conversation. Some patients are on the edge of aggression, and using the correct body language can make a difference in their demeanor.

31.

B. If the patient will not sign the refusal-of-care form, have a family member sign, stating that the patient refused to sign. A police officer or bystander can also sign. The person signing is witnessing that the patient refused to sign the document but is not signing the refusal for the patient. This person is a witness for your protection because the patient could state later that he wanted to be treated and for that reason did not sign the report.

32.

B. Acute abdominal pain is not a sign of respiratory distress. Restlessness and agitation are signs that the brain is not getting enough oxygen. Accessory muscle use is a sign of inadequate breathing; the intercostal muscles and the diaphragm are used to try to force more air into the lungs. Incomprehensible or mumbled speech could indicate that the brain is not receiving enough oxygen.

33.

B. It is not important to determine the cause of a patient's breathing difficulty except for a trauma patient. Expose and inspect the trauma patient's chest and treat accordingly. The EMT as should provide positive pressure ventilation whenever in doubt as to the patient's ventilatory status. Patients with breathing difficulty are considered priority patients.

34.

D. Decreased wheezing is frequently, although not always, an indication of patient improvement, but if it is combined with a deterioration in the patient's mental status, it could indicate severe bronchospasm with less air movement. Be sure to assess not only for the abnormal sounds but also for normal breath sounds. If the wheezing is decreasing but normal breath sounds have not returned or are barely audible, the patient's constriction has likely worsened. This patient will need to be ventilated.

35.

C. Increased oxygenation frequently improves cerebral oxygenation. Improved cerebral oxygenation results in improvement in the patient's mental status, especially a reduction in restlessness and anxiety because the mental status is directly related to the hypoxic state.

36.

A. This patient has late signs of respiratory distress. Cyanosis and tachycardia are ominous signs of severe respiratory distress. This patient must be immediately ventilated with positive pressure ventilations. This patient is a priority patient and should be transported immediately. Continue your assessment while en route to the hospital. You should also consider advanced life support backup with priority patients.

37.

A. You should provide positive pressure ventilation immediately. The patient is making efforts to breathe; however, breathing is not effective. Never withhold oxygen from a patient who complains of breathing difficulty. Oxygen by nasal cannula or nonrebreather mask is not sufficient for this patient; ventilate him.

38.

C. The patient should be instructed to hold his breath for as long as possible after the administration and then exhale slowly through pursed lips. This increases the deposit of the medication deep in the bronchiole. The canister must be shaken because the medication is in suspension and needs to be mixed in the canister. Depress the canister as the patient begins to inhale deeply.

39.

B. Croup, a childhood condition, is characterized by a high-pitched sound from swelling of the larynx. Exposing the child to the cool night air frequently diminishes its signs and symptoms.

40.

C. The most common cause of mechanical failure is related to batteries. Ensure that they are properly maintained to prevent this type of equipment failure.

41.

D. When a patient is in cardiac arrest for more than 4 to 5 minutes, you should first perform five cycles of CPR prior to attaching the AED. The five cycles of CPR will provide the necessary oxygen and nutrients to the heart and improve the chance that the defibrillation will be successful.

42.

A. When the patient has taken more than three nitroglycerin tablets prior to your arrival, refrain from administering any additional doses, as you would if the systolic blood pressure were below 100 mmHg, or the patient has a head injury. Headache is a common side effect of nitroglycerin.

43.

C. Because nitroglycerin is a potent vasodilator, hypotension is a potential side effect. The heart rate could increase due to the vasodilation and reduced volume to the left side of the heart. Bradycardia and dyspnea are not common side effects.

44.

A. To deliver nitroglycerin spray, depress the container once, delivering one short spray. The nitroglycerin spray container is metered and delivers only the correct dose each time it is depressed.

45.

D. Diseases of the heart and blood vessels represent the number one killer of people in the United States today.

46.

A. Approximately 20 percent of heart attacks are painless or silent, that is, with no associated pain. You must rely on other signs and symptoms of a heart attack to help you determine that the patient is having a silent one.

47.

C. You should remove the nitroglycerin patch and wipe the area clean with a cloth. Be sure to wear gloves so that you do not absorb the nitroglycerin through your skin. Remove the patch and place the AED pads before defibrillating the patient. If the nitroglycerin patch is not removed, the current from the defibrillator can melt the plastic and cause a fire.

48.

C. External defibrillators are categorized into two main types: manual defibrillator (requires extensive skills to operate) and automatic. There are two types of automatic defibrillators, the automatic and semi-automatic. The implantable defibrillator is categorized as an internal defibrillator.

49.

D. This patient's breathing is shallow and slow (bradypnea). This inadequate breathing must be assisted by positive pressure ventilation immediately.

If the patient is breathing adequately, you should administer oxygen by nonrebreather mask at 15 lpm.

50.

A. Nitroglycerin causes coronary artery vasodilation. Blood vessels in other parts of the body also dilate. The body could compensate for this by increasing the pulse rate slightly. The patient's blood pressure will most likely decrease. Nitroglycerin decreases the heart's workload.

51.

D. The ratio of chest compressions to ventilation for one- and two-person CPR for the adult patient is 30 compressions to 2 ventilations. In the infant and child, the ratio of 15 compressions to 2 ventilations is acceptable when performing two-person CPR.

52.

D. A high level of sugar in the blood is called *hyperglycemia*. A low blood sugar level in the blood is called *hypoglycemia*. When insulin production is insufficient, the sugar cannot leave the blood and enter the body cells. This causes an increase in the blood sugar level.

53.

D. The hypoglycemic patient who has an altered mental status should be placed on the side. This position helps to protect the airway if the patient vomits. All of the other positions can cause secretions to be aspirated into the airway due to the patient's inability to pro-tect it.

54.

B. A stiff neck is a late sign of neurological deficit that has resulted from a nontraumatic brain injury. There are many different signs and symptoms of neurological deficit, depending on the location of the brain injury.

55.

D. The recovery phase of a seizure is the *postictal state*. During this period of time, the patient's mental status progressively improves. The patient can present with a severe headache or temporary hemiparesis.

56.
B. The aura is the first phase, and if present, involves some type of sensory perception by the patient. The second or tonic phase occurs when the patient's muscles contract and tense and the patient exhibits extreme muscular rigidity with arching of the back. This is followed by the occurrence of convulsions, or the clonic phase. The last phase is the postictal state or the recovery period, which lasts from 10 to 30 minutes.

57.
A. A transient ischemic attack generally subsides within 5 to 10 minutes, the signs and symptoms are identical to the presentation of a stroke patient, but the patient recovers without any neurological deficit.

58.
C. Strokes most often affect elderly patients with a history of hardening of the arteries (atherosclerosis) or hypertension (high blood pressure). More than half of stroke patients die, and many others suffer permanent neurological damage.

59.
B. *Syncope* occurs when a temporary lack of blood and oxygen flow to the brain occurs over a short time period. It commonly happens when the patient is standing. When the patient assumes a supine position, he improves rapidly.

60.
B. In anaphylaxis, the two primary body systems affected are the respiratory and circulatory systems as a result of bronchoconstriction and peripheral vasodilatation.

61.
A. Epinephrine works almost immediately; however, its effective duration is short, approximately 10 to 20 minutes. Because of this short time, you should transport immediately and consider advanced life support backup.

62.
C. Do not administer epinephrine to the patient who is suffering a mild reaction unless you are directed to do so by medical direction. This patient is elderly and could suffer serious side effects from the administration of epinephrine. The adverse side effects do not outweigh the benefits for this patient's current condition as described.

63.
A. An *allergen* is a substance that enters the body by ingestion, injection, inhalation, or contact and triggers an allergic reaction.

64.
A. Activated charcoal is the medication of choice to use for ingested poisonings. Activated charcoal works by absorbing the poison and thus prevents the body from doing so.

65.
B. A patient who has acute abdominal pain and is in shock (hypoperfusion) should be placed in a supine position with the feet elevated. This position helps to increase perfusion to the brain and other vital organs.

66.
C. The 34-year-old is middle aged and should tolerate cold better than the young and old. This person is walking briskly, which increases body temperature through muscle contractions. Certain medications and alcohol decrease a person's ability to tolerate a cold environment. A wet person loses more heat than a dry person.

67.
A. You should wash the bite area with a mild soap and water, being careful not to aggressively scrub. The injection site should be placed slightly lower than the level of the patient's heart. Never lacerate the injection site to try to evacuate the poison; this could further complicate the patient's recovery and does not remove toxins. Tourniquets should not be used in a snake bite injury. Some protocols allow the use of restricting bands; consult your local medical direction.

68.
D. Simply stated, *reasonable force* is the minimum amount of force required to keep a patient from injuring himself or others.

69.

D. To prevent supine hypotension syndrome in the patient who is near full term of her pregnancy, place her in a lateral recumbent or a sitting position. If the patient must lie flat, place her on her left side or raise her right hip. If placed in the supine position, the weight of the uterus and fetus presses on the inferior vena cava and causes inadequate blood return to the heart, causing poor cardiac output.

70.

D. The placenta must be transported to the hospital for examination by a physician. The physician will then determine whether the delivery was complete. Normal blood loss after delivery is up to 500 cc and is well tolerated. The placenta usually delivers within 10 minutes of the fetus and almost always within 20 minutes. Do not apply pressure to the infant's fontanel; the soft depressed area of the infant's head.

71.

B. The placenta usually delivers within 10 to 20 minutes following delivery. Do not delay transport while waiting for its delivery. Transport the placenta in a plastic bag with the patient. This allows a physician to examine it to confirm that the placenta delivery was complete.

72.

B. The umbilical cord should be cut after the pulsations in the cord cease. Two clamps are positioned on the cord before cutting it.

73.

B. The fingertips of the gloved hand are positioned on the bony part of the infant's head to prevent an explosive delivery.

74.

A. The brachial artery is located in the upper arm; arterial bleeding is bright red and spurts with each heart contraction. The femoral artery is located in the upper leg. The cephalic vein is located in the upper arm; however, bleeding from a vein is dark red and steady. The peroneal vein is located in the lower leg.

75.

C. Severe bleeding that is life threatening should be controlled during the primary assessment. Control severe bleeding after you secure the airway, breathing, and circulation. Often, bleeding control can be accomplished simultaneously with airway and breathing management.

76.

C. When treating a closed soft tissue injury like a large hematoma, you must first take BSI precautions. Next, ensure that the patient has an open airway and is breathing adequately. If the patient is not breathing adequately or has a closed airway, stop and correct the airway or breathing problem. After ensuring that the airway is adequate, quickly treat for shock. After treating for shock, you should next splint any painful, swollen, or deformed extremities.

77.

B. You should cut the shirt away from the adhered portion. Never remove adhered clothing. This can cause extreme pain and further damage the burn site. Never apply ointments of any kind to burns; most often these ointments must be removed at the hospital.

78.

D. Never attempt to break or drain blisters from a burn; doing so will likely introduce contaminants and increase the possibility of infection.

79.

A. A bandage holds in place a dressing (2 × 2, 4 × 4) in size, which should be sterile and placed directly on the wound. Common bandages include self-adhering, gauze rolls, and triangular.

80.

D. When blood soaks through the original dressings, you should apply additional ones over the original ones. Removing the original dressings aggravates the wound and increases the bleeding. Tourniquets should be applied only as a last resort. A loose tourniquet acts as a restricting band and can cause the pressure in the blood vessel to increase, thus increasing the bleeding.

answers & rationales

81.
D. Leaving the fingertips or toes exposed after bandaging allows for the assessment of circulation by examining skin color and temperature. Bandages must not impair circulation distal to an injury.

82.
D. Your first action should be to manually secure the object to reduce the likelihood that it will cause further injury or become dislodged. Next, expose the wound site, and than control the bleeding from around the object. Last, use a bulky dressing to help stabilize the object. Never remove any object that is embedded in the chest.

83.
C. The anterior bone of the lower leg is called the *tibia*. The posterior bone is called the *fibula*.

84.
B. Splints should be appropriately padded to prevent pressure. Perform only one alignment attempt if the distal pulse is absent in an extremity. Any jewelry around the injury site should be removed. *Never* intentionally return broken bone ends to beneath the skin.

85.
D. The EMT should *never* ask the patient to move in an attempt to determine the anatomical location of a potential spinal injury. This can cause irreversible spinal cord injury. Impaired breathing can result from damage at the level of the cervical spine. Soft tissue injury of the head and neck are frequent indications of possible spinal injury.

86.
D. A helmet should be left in place if you can properly immobilize the head because it prevents head movement. The helmet should be removed if it interferes with the assessment or management of the airway or breathing. If the helmet does not fit well and allows excessive head movement to occur, it should be removed.

87.
C. The EMT must quickly and continuously irrigate the patient's eyes when dealing with eye burns. Do not use any irrigate other than saline or water. Continue flushing the eyes during transport. Remove contact lenses to prevent trapping chemical agents under them.

88.
A. Cyanosis (blue color) indicates that your pediatric patient is in decompensated respiratory failure, and positive pressure ventilation must be performed. All other distracters are early signs of respiratory distress in the pediatric patient.

89.
B. Weak or absent peripheral pulses indicate poor circulation, which indicates hypoperfusion (shock). Other signs are rapid respiratory rate; pale, cool, and clammy skin; decreased mental status; and prolonged capillary refill in the patient under six years of age.

90.
B. Neglect occurs when the caregiver provides insufficient respect or attention to an individual—such as child or an elderly person—for whom the caregiver is responsible. Physical abuse occurs when improper or excessive action injures or harms a person.

91.
D. It is dangerous to accelerate while in a curve. You should carefully and gradually accelerate after exiting the curve. You should brake or decelerate prior to entering the curve; you should only drive as fast as feels comfortable. You should enter a curve on the outside or highest part.

92.
C. To protect yourself and the patient from debris, cover using a tarpaulin or heavy blanket. Even the most careful spreader operator cannot keep debris from becoming projectiles. A rapid extrication should be performed if the patient's condition re-

quires it or there is a real threat to the well-being of the rescue personnel. Giving your protective clothing to the patient will not protect you.

93.

B. Simple access is best described as access that does not require the use of tools.

94.

A. Your immediate role as the EMT who responds to a possible hazardous material spill is to cordon off the area and evacuate all bystanders. Do not approach the site even if patients are visible. Move bystanders uphill and upwind. Do not approach the site to try to identify the type of cargo being transported.

95.

B. Your initial role as the first EMT on the scene of a MCI is as the incident manager until the designated incident manager relieves you.

96.

B. A patient with burns without airway problems should be tagged yellow—second priority. Red is the highest priority for airway problems, severe bleeding, and shock. Green is a low priority for minor burns, minor injuries, and walking wounded. Black is the lowest priority for obviously dead patients.

97.

C. A nasogastric tube is indicated in the infant or child patient when you are unable to provide positive pressure ventilation due to gastric distention. It is also indicated when an unresponsive patient is at risk of vomiting or developing gastric distention.

98.

A. A stylet is commonly used to facilitate the placement of the endotracheal tube. Ventilation of a patient with an endotracheal tube in place does not require the use of a mask. The endotracheal tube provides a direct route to the patient's lungs for ventilation. In addition to the stylet, the following are needed to intubate a patient: endotracheal tube, water-soluble lubricant, 10 cc syringe, endotracheal tube securing device, towels or padding, and a stethoscope.

99.

C. The stylet is used to alter the shape of the endotracheal tube and to make the tube stiffer. Be sure that the stylet does not extend beyond the end of the endotracheal tube. This could cause damage to the soft tissues of the airway.

100.

B. The right mainstem bronchus, not the left mainstem, is more likely to be intubated. Complications in addition to those listed are bradycardia, hypertension, vomiting, and laryngospasm.

101.

A. Touching or stimulating the patient's vocal cords or epiglottis can result in laryngospasm of the vocal cords. They will close completely and not allow air to pass through but will eventually relax and allow air to pass through. Positive pressure ventilation is necessary if the cords do not relax immediately.

102.

C. Bradycardia in the infant or child is an early sign of hypoxia. If the heart rate drops below 80 beats/minute in the infant or 60 in the child, stop the intubation attempt and hyperoxygenate the patient. Then reattempt the intubation.

103.

A. The technique is called *digital intubation. Oral intubation* is placement of an endotracheal tube through the mouth. Technically, it is a digital intubation that is placed orally.

104.

D. The open wound to the chest is an immediate life threat. You must occlude it with your gloved hand and then place an occlusive dressing over it. You must inspect the entire thorax to look for other possible stab wounds.

105.

B. The cyanosis is an indication of poor ventilation and inadequate oxygen exchange. The pale, cool, clammy skin and low pulse oximeter reading is an indication of hypoxia. If there were inadequate tissue perfusion or shock, you would expect to have a weak and thready radial pulse and a narrow pulse pressure.

106.

C. Your next step in emergency care of the patient is to begin bag-valve-mask ventilation. The patient has a respiratory rate of 42/minute and shallow rise of the chest, both indications of inadequate breathing. Ventilate the patient at 10 to 12 times per minute and be sure to attach supplemental oxygen to the bag-valve-mask device.

107.

A. You should call for a specialized rescue team without delay and await its arrival. When you encounter a scene calling for specialized rescue, you should try to stabilize the scene and protect the patient without putting yourself or him in danger. In this case, the patient is atop the vehicle and somewhat safe.

108.

D. This patient sustained an open (compound) fracture to the left distal femur. The femur is the large bone that is located above the knee (patella). The fracture is open because it punctured through the skin.

109.

C. Bleeding from a vein usually appears to be dark red and flows steadily. Arterial bleeding presents as bright red bleeding that spurts from the wound with each heart beat. Capillary bleeding is dark red and slowly oozes from the wound. Bleeding from arterioles is part of arterial bleeding.

110.

C. You should manage this patient's injuries by first applying direct pressure to the extremity, the site of bleeding. Then elevate the extremity and apply a cold pack to the site. Most bleeding injuries can be controlled with these steps. A tourniquet is rarely needed to control bleeding and is a last resort effort.

111.

D. Gurgling indicates that the patient has a liquid substance in the airway which must immediately be cleared by suction before the patient aspirates it into his lungs. After suctioning the patient, you should begin bag-valve-mask ventilation. Supplemental oxygen must be connected to the ventilation device.

112.

B. The patient most likely has a spinal cord injury and distributive shock from massive vasodilation of the vessels below the injury. In hypovolemic shock, the blood pressure is low, the heart rate is elevated, and the skin is pale, cool, and clammy. In a vasogenic shock, the blood pressure is low, the heart rate is low, and the skin is warm, flushed, and dry below the site of the injury.

113.

D. A *contact burn* occurs from contact with a hot object such as the exhaust pipe of the vehicle. A *flame burn* occurs when there is contact with an open flame. A *flash burn* is a type of burn that occurs from a flash flame; it is usually associated with a gas or liquid that quickly ignites. "Radiant" is not a type of burn.

114.

A. The hand must be splinted in a position of function. This is achieved by placing a roll of bandage in the hand and having the patient extend the fingers. Failing to use this position can cause further injury to the hand.

115.

D. The best indicator of improvement or deterioration of a patient with a head injury is the level of consciousness. The Glasgow Coma Scale assigns numerical values for monitoring a patient's level of consciousness. A higher number indicates good brain function; a lower number indicates poor brain function.

116.

A. An unresponsive medical patient should be placed in a lateral recumbent position to protect his airway and keep him from aspirating secretions and vomitus. However, because the patient in this case requires ventilation, he must be placed in a supine position. It would be extremely difficult to ventilate a patient who is on his side. You must constantly monitor the airway and have suction available when the patient is in a supine position.

117.
D. The best treatment for an amputated body part is to wrap it in a saline-moistened, sterile dressing and place it in a plastic bag. Place the plastic bag on ice packs or ice with a towel separating the ice and bag to keep the body part cool. Never place the body part directly on ice because this can cause the tissue to freeze, which damages it. Label the bag and transport it without delay.

118.
D. Turning off the ignition eliminates the majority of the electrical hazards. Although many departments disconnect the battery cables, some vehicles can still present dangers until the ignition is switched off. Disconnecting other electrical wires is a danger to you and others on the scene.

119.
A. You should apply a sterile dressing moistened with sterile saline. Then you should keep the dressing and the exposed organs from drying by covering the dressing with an occlusive dressing. It is best to keep the organs moist.

120.
C. Based in the mechanism of injury, you should first establish inline spine stabilization. You would then perform a jaw thrust to open the airway.

121.
D. You should cover the eye with a moist, sterile dressing to prevent the injured tissue from adhering to the dressing. Never apply pressure to an injured eye. Be sure to transport any avulsed tissue to the hospital in case it can be reattached. Preserve the part by wrapping it in a moist sterile dressing and keeping it cool.

122.
C. In a tension pneumothorax, breath sounds will be absent on the injured side and decreased on the uninjured side. The air on the injured side forces the mediastinum to shift, compressing the chest cavity on the uninjured side, interfering with the inflation of the lung on the uninjured side.

123.
D. Clear fluid, blood, or blood-tinged fluid draining from the ear can indicate a skull fracture. You should place a loose sterile dressing across the opening of the ear to absorb the fluids. Never pack or exert any pressure to restrict or tamponade the leaking fluid.

124.
C. The patient's breathing is inadequate; thus, she needs to be ventilated immediately with a bag-valve-mask device. You cannot insert an oropharyngeal air because she is still awake and responsive.

125.
B. A patient who presents with a sudden onset of numbness, tingling, weakness, or paralysis to the extremities; slurred speech; confusion or altered mental status; or facial droop can be having a stroke.

126.
C. Arm strength, facial droop, and speech are highly predictive of a stroke and should be assessed in any patient suspected of having had one. Most EMS systems use Cincinnati Prehospital Stroke Scale (CPSS) or the Los Angeles Prehospital Stroke Scale (LAPSS) when assessing patients for stroke.

127.
D. Your next immediate action is to administer oxygen and then to assess the patient's circulation (pulse and perfusion status). He is complaining of chest discomfort upon your arrival, so you have already determined his mental status, airway, and breathing status. You need to assess the circulation to complete the primary assessment.

128.
C. The red blotchy skin, respiratory distress, hoarseness, stridor, and elevated heart rate all indicate a severe allergic reaction or anaphylaxis.

129.
B. You should have the mother continue to hold the child in her lap and provide the oxygen via a blow-by method by holding the oxygen mask near the child's face. By removing the child from the mother's

lap or forcing the oxygen to his face, you will only increase his anxiety and the workload to breathe.

130.

A. Approximately 50 percent of the patients who receive prehospital defibrillation will deteriorate back into ventricular fibrillation. Thus, it is extremely important to get an advanced life support unit to respond to administer medications to help keep the patient from going back into ventricular fibrillation.

131.

C. If the cardiac arrest is witnessed once and you have verified pulselessness and apnea, you should next immediately attach the advanced external defibrillator (AED) and begin rhythm analysis. If the arrest was not witnessed and an estimated 4 to 5 minutes have passed since the patient went into cardiac arrest, you would complete five cycles of CPR before attaching the AED.

132.

C. The shockable rhythms are ventricular fibrillation and ventricular tachycardia. A patient can be in ventricular tachycardia and still have a pulse and be alert. Thus, it is extremely important to determine pulselessness and apnea prior to applying the AED.

133.

A. The prescription of Humulin suggested that the patient is a diabetic. He is exhibiting signs and symptoms of hypoglycemia: pale, cool, clammy skin; altered mental status; and tachycardia. Because he is still awake and able to talk, your next immediate action should be to administer one tube of oral glucose.

134.

D. Hypoxia causes the patient to become agitated and restless. As the carbon dioxide level increases in the blood, the patient becomes confused and disoriented.

135.

B. The patient is in status epilepticus, which is a dire emergency. Because he is unable to breathe effectively during a seizure, it is necessary to insert an airway and begin bag-valve-mask ventilation. You

cannot administer oral glucose because the pateint is not awake or able to swallow it.

136.

D. The patient is a candidate for nitroglycerin administration; however, you would administer oxygen as part of the primary assessment because the pale, cool skin may be an indication of hypoxia.

137.

D. The skin is red and warm due to the systemic vasodilation. When the vessels in the skin dilate, they fill with the warm red blood, producing flushed and warm skin.

138.

B. You have just assessed the patient's responsiveness. You should immediately open the airway and assess the respiratory status. When you have done that, assess the ciruclation.

139.

A. A *deficit* is an abnormality. Neurologic deficits can be cognitive; that is, they involve the thinking process. Sensory deficits involve the ability to feel a touch, pain, or a vibration. Motor deficits involve movement.

140.

B. The patient is breathing inadequately; thus, he needs to be ventilated immediately. You cannot administer oral glucose due to the altered mental status.

141.

C. A *convulsion* is the jerky movement caused by alternating muscular rigidity and relaxation. A convulsion is only one sign of a seizure, which is the overall condition and might not present with convulsions.

142.

A. The hives (urticaria) and itching (pruritis) are due to the leaking capillaries. The red, warm skin is due to the vasodilation. The hypotension and tachycardia are due to the vasodilation and loss of fluid from the leaking capillaries.

143.

C. An increasing heart rate from within a normal range to outside a normal range indicates that the ventilation is likely ineffective and the patient is continuing to become more hypoxic. A narcotic overdose would cause the heart rate to decrease.

144.

B. Ventolin is a beta 2 specific agonist drug that produces bronchodilation. The wheezing is due to bronchoconstriction and inflammation inside of the airway. There is no indication for the administration of nitroglycerin. The EMT cannot administer digitalis or coumadin.

145.

C. The patient who complains of the "worst headache" is usually experiencing a hemorrhagic stroke. Embolic and thrombotic strokes are typically associated with headache; however, it is usually mild to moderate.

146.

B. The patient who exhibited signs and symptoms of a stroke that disappear within 1 hour of the onset has had a transient ischemic attack. The patient recovers completely and has no residual neurologic deficit.

147.

C. The patient is still experiencing the anaphylactic reaction. If the patient has a second epinephrine autoinjector, contact medical direction for permission to administer the second dose.

148.

A. Insulin is a hormone that is secreted by the beta cells in the Islets of Langerhans. It attaches to a receptor site on the cell membrane and opens a protein channel that allows the glucose to be carried into the cell by a protein carrier. Glucose can enter the cell at a rate of about 10 times faster when insulin is available. If insulin is not available, the glucose will begin to accumulate in the blood, resulting in hyperglycemia. If too much insulin is in the blood, the glucose will rapidly enter the cells and little will be left in the blood, causing hypoglycemia.

149.

D. Nitroglycerin cannot be administered if the patient has taken Viagra, Cialis, or any other drug for erectile dysfunction. Nitroglycerin is contraindicated and could produce serious side effects if administered.

150.

A. The patient is most likely experiencing hyperventilation syndrome. These patients commonly complain that they cannot breathe and are having chest discomfort. Other symptoms include lightheadedness, dizziness, and sometimes actual fainting. The best treatment is to remove the patient from the stimulus that is making him anxious and to calm him down. Do not have the patient breath into a paper bag or an oxygen mask that is not connected to oxygen. That is a dangerous practice.

Appendix: Correlation of Success for the EMT to the National Registry of EMTs 2009 Practice Analysis Test Plan

NREMT Practice Analysis Test Plan: Sections with Task	Correlation to Success for the EMT
Section: Airway, Respiration, and Ventilation	
Task: Airway Management	Section 2: Airway, Respiration and Ventilation Section 3: Patient Assessment Section 6: Infants and Children
Task: Ventilation	Section 2: Airway, Respiration and Ventilation Section 3: Patient Assessment Section 6: Infants and Children
Task: Respiratory Distress	Section 2: Airway, Respiration and Ventilation Section 3: Patient Assessment Section 6: Infants and Children
Task: Respiratory Failure	Section 2: Airway, Respiration and Ventilation Section 3: Patient Assessment Section 6: Infants and Children
Task: Respiratory Arrest	Section 2: Airway, Respiration and Ventilation Section 3: Patient Assessment Section 6: Infants and Children
Task: Upper Airway Respiratory Emergencies	Section 2: Airway, Respiration and Ventilation Section 3: Patient Assessment Section 4: Medical/Gynecology/Obstetrics – Respiratory Emergencies Section 6: Infants and Children

Task: Lower Airway Respiratory Emergencies

Section 2: Airway, Respiration and Ventilation
Section 3: Patient Assessment
Section 4: Medical/Gynecology/Obstetrics –
Respiratory Emergencies
Section 6: Infants and Children

Section: Cardiology and Resuscitation

Task: Chest Pain

Section 4: Medical/Gynecology/Obstetrics –
General Pharmacology and
Cardiovascular Emergencies

Task: Cardiac Rhythm Disturbance

Section 4: Medical/Gynecology/Obstetrics –
Cardiovascular Emergencies

Task: Cardiac Arrest

Section 4: Medical/Gynecology/Obstetrics –
Cardiovascular Emergencies

Task: Stroke-like Symptoms

Section 4: Medical/Gynecology/Obstetrics –
Stroke

Task: Post-resuscitation Care

Section 4: Medical/Gynecology/Obstetrics –
Cardiovascular Emergencies

Task: Hypotension/Hypertension from Cardiovascular Care

Section 4: Medical/Gynecology/Obstetrics –
Cardiovascular Emergencies

Section: Trauma

Task: Bleeding

Section 3: Patient Assessment
Section 5: Trauma

Task: Chest Trauma

Section 3: Patient Assessment
Section 5: Trauma

Task: Abdominal/GU Trauma

Section 3: Patient Assessment
Section 5: Trauma

Task: Orthopedic Trauma

Section 3: Patient Assessment
Section 5: Trauma

Task: Soft Tissue

Section 3: Patient Assessment
Section 5: Trauma

Task: Head/Neck/Face/Spine

Section 3: Patient Assessment
Section 5: Trauma

Task: Multisystem Trauma

Section 3: Patient Assessment
Section 5: Trauma

Section:
Medical/Obstetrics/Gynecology

Task: Neurologic Emergencies

Section 4: Medical/Gynecology/Obstetrics – Diabetes/Altered Mental Status, and Seizures and Syncope

Task: Abdominal Disorders

Section 4: Medical/Gynecology/Obstetrics – Acute Abdominal Pain

Task: Immunology

Section 4: Medical/Gynecology/Obstetrics – Allergic Reaction/Anaphylaxis

Task: Infectious Disease

Section 1: Preparatory

Task: Endocrine Disorders

Section 4: Medical/Gynecology/Obstetrics – Diabetes/Altered Mental Status

Task: Psychiatric

Section 4: Medical/Gynecology/Obstetrics – Psychiatric Emergencies

Task: Toxicology

Section 4: Medical/Gynecology/Obstetrics – Poisoning/Overdose Emergencies

Task: Gynecology

Section 4: Medical/Gynecology/Obstetrics – Obstetrics and Gynecology

Task: Obstetrics

Section 4: Medical/Gynecology/Obstetrics – Obstetrics and Gynecology

Section: EMS Operations

Task: Maintain Vehicle and Equipment Readiness

Section 7: Operations

Task: Operate Emergency Vehicles

Section 7: Operations

Task: Provide Scene Leadership

Section 1: Preparatory
Section 3: Patient Assessment
Section 7: Operations

Task: Resolve an Emergency Incident

Section 7: Operations

Task: Provide Emotional Support

Section 1: Preparatory
Section 3: Patient Assessment

Task: Maintain Medical/Legal Standards

Section 1: Preparatory

Task: Maintain Community Relations

Section 1: Preparatory

Task: Provide Administrative Support

Section 1: Preparatory

Task: Enhance Professional Development

Section 1: Preparatory

Index

Notes

Notes

Notes

Notes

Notes

Notes

Notes

Notes

Notes

Notes

Notes

Notes

Notes

Notes

Notes

Notes

Notes

Notes

Notes

Notes